Problems in Cardiology

Problems in Practice Series

Series Editors : J.Fry K.Williams M.Lancaster-Smith

Problems
in
Cardiology

Christopher F. P. Wharton
MA, DM(Oxon), FRCP

Consultant Physician
Farnborough, Orpington and Sevenoaks Hospitals, Kent

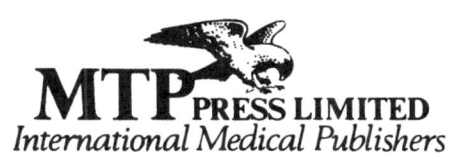

MTP PRESS LIMITED
International Medical Publishers

Published by
MTP Press Limited
Falcon House
Lancaster, England

First published 1981

ISBN-13: 978-94-011-7211-0   e-ISBN-13: 978-94-011-7209-7
DOI: 10.1007/978-94-011-7209-7

Typesetting by Swiftpages Ltd, Liverpool and

Trowbridge

Contents

Preface

Over several years working in a district general hospital as a physician with a cardiological interest, the common problems in this field are clearer. This knowledge has come through normal out-patient clinic referrals, care of in-patients, and by working in a domiciliary consultative capacity.

The problems that concern family physicians nowadays are somewhat different from the problems of two or three decades ago. The accent now is very much on the implications of hypertensive and ischaemic heart disease. Rheumatic fever is rarely seen, though its sequelae may still be discovered. Hence the approach of this book is to the common problems of today in family practice, and the book is not intended to be a reference text book of cardiology. It does not include references because it has been written from personal experience gained from the treatment and management of patients with common cardiac problems.

It is hoped that it will be of value primarily to family physicians because it has been written in an attempt to fill a need as measured by the problems that are referred to specialists in the cardiological field. It may prove of value to those medical students and nurses who wish to consider medical problems in a practical way, that is from the ways that cardiac problems present in practice.

C. F. P. Wharton
Farnborough, Kent

Series Foreword

This series of books is designed to help general practitioners. So are other books. What is unusual in this instance is their collective authorship; they are written by specialists working at district general hospitals. The writers derive their own experience from a range of cases less highly selected than those on which textbooks are traditionally based. They are also in a good position to pick out topics which they see creating difficulties for the practitioners of their district, whose personal capacities are familiar to them; and to concentrate on contexts where mistakes are most likely to occur. They are all well-accustomed to working in consultation.

All the authors write from hospital experience and from the viewpoint of their specialty. There are, therefore, matters important to family practice which should be sought not within this series, but elsewhere. Within the series much practical and useful advice is to be found with which the general practitioner can compare his existing performance and build in new ideas and improved techniques.

These books are attractively produced and I recommend them.

J. P. Horder OBE
President, The Royal College
of General Practitioners

9

1 Presenting symptoms – chest pain

Skin – Intercostal muscles and muscles attached to the chest wall – Ribs and spine – Costo-chondral junctions – Pleura and diaphragmatic pleura – The pericardium – The myocardium – The aorta – The oesophagus – Anxiety and cardiac neurosis

Patients will describe a wide variety of chest pains in the consulting room or surgery and of the symptoms with which a doctor may be confronted, chest pain is one of the most important to assess. The possible implications of chest pains are obvious but it must be remembered when dealing with the symptom, that uppermost in the patient's mind is whether the pain may signify either coronary artery disease or lung cancer. The former condition should be to the fore of the doctor's thoughts and it is with this in mind that the types of chest pain are considered in this chapter in an attempt to aid the diagnosis or exclusion of coronary artery disease as a cause of pain. A few minutes of careful questioning by the doctor will determine in most cases the nature of the pain and an opinion may be formed as to whether or not it is cardiac pain.

The *main structures of the thorax* which may give rise to pain should be remembered. These are:

The origins of chest pain

(1) The skin,
(2) Intercostal muscles and muscles attached to the chest wall,
(3) Ribs and the spine,
(4) Costo-chondral junctions,
(5) Pleura and diaphragmatic pleura,
(6) The pericardium,

11

(7) The myocardium,
(8) The aorta,
(9) The oesophagus,
(10) Anxiety about various thoracic structures and cardiac neurosis.

(1) Skin

Causes of pain are obvious, infections in the form of boils and abscesses are self-evident. Shingles infecting the intercostal nerves may not be evident, vesicles of the skin do not appear until a few days after the pain has appeared. Post-herpetic neuralgia is another important cause of pain and is notoriously difficult to treat.

(2) Intercostal muscles and muscles attached to the chest wall

Pain originating from thoracic wall musculature and inter-costal muscles often follows a history of trauma, lifting or twisting. The pain is very often associated with tenderness on palpation of the site of the pain, reproducing a mild type of the discomfort complained of, or can be provoked by twisting the thorax.

Intercostal myositis or myalgia is usually of viral origin associated with a typical viral infection producing fever, head-aches and aching limbs, sore throat and perhaps abdominal or pleuritic pain. The common organism is a Coxsackie B virus (Bornholm's disease).

(3) Ribs and the spine

Osteoarthritis of the dorsal or thoracic spine and disc lesions by nerve compression may produce anterior chest pain radiat-ing to the left arm, and it should be remembered that disorders which involve deep afferent fibres of the left upper thoracic region can cause pain in the chest and left arm. So a history of spinal problems or cervical spondylosis is extremely important, and pain may be reproduced by extreme movement of the neck. The diagnosis may be supported by depressed or absent reflexes in the arm of the affected side.

The ribs are an important site of pain. Trauma causing fractures, cracks or bruises is common and involvement of the ribs by tumours (mammary or bronchial), or secondaries, causing pathological fractures is not infrequently seen, e.g. myelomatosis or carcinomatosis.

(4) Costo-chondral junctions

The commonest cause of costo-chondral pain is a low grade costo-chondritis and this is a common cause of anterior chest wall pain. This may be evidenced by swelling, redness and is tender to pressure (Tietze's syndrome).

(5) Pleura and diaphragmatic pleura

Pleuritic pain is characteristically sharp and is provoked on the inspiratory phase of respiration or at the extreme inspiratory point. Rarely, there is tenderness over it. If the diaphragmatic pleura is involved, the pain may radiate to the shoulder tip. It may be caused by inflammation of the pleura or by underlying pulmonary disease, infarction, pneumonia or tumour.

(6) The pericardium

Pericardial pain is also sharp and often severe. It may be central, retrosternal pain but is often in part pleuritic and is provoked or relieved by change of posture, such as lying or sitting up and turning on the side. If due to a viral pericarditis the prodromal symptoms of viral infection may be noted.

(7) The myocardium

It is most important of all to know the exact nature of myocardial pain. Pain originating from damage to the myocardium due to either ischaemia or infarction is characteristic, though is occasionally atypical and then difficult to interpret. The pain is central and retrosternal and may radiate to the throat and the arms, the left more commonly than the right. As explained above, this distribution and radiation is not peculiar to cardiac pain, the precipitating and relieving factors are enormously important. Anginal type pain may be:

(i) Provoked by *exercise or exertion* and *relieved by resting.*

(ii) Provoked by sudden change of *air temperature,* e.g. going out into *cold air* first thing in the day.

(iii) Provoked by *meals,* particularly *exertion after food.*

(iv) Provoked by emotional *stress* or excitement.

(v) Anginal pain is usually *relieved by Trinitrin* (GTN) quickly.

Anginal pain and infarction pain

Cardiac pain that persists at rest for more than fifteen minutes is probably associated with impending infarction, and angina of effort, becoming more and more frequent until it occurs at rest, may herald infarction (crescendo angina).

Angina decubitus

There is a particular form of angina which occurs at rest in bed at night when the patient is flat. This is angina decubitus, presumably due to increased venous return causing an increase in pre-load which puts extra demand on myocardial function. Prinzmetal's angina also occurs at rest and is associated with ventricular dysrhythmias, and ST elevation is seen on e.c.g.

The essential quality of cardiac pain is that it is crushing, squeezing, vice-like, or like a heavy weight or pressure on the sternum. The patient may sometimes demonstrate this by applying pressure with the palm of his hand on the sternum, or squeeze both pectoral areas toward the centre with the palms of his hands. This is very characteristic.

Cardiac pain is often associated with a feeling of ill-being such as faintness, weakness or light-headedness and sweating.

(8) The aorta

Pain from a dissection of the aorta is like pain from cardiac infarction but is if anything more severe, may be felt in the back and is more persistent, with marked disturbance of the patient's general condition, producing hypotension, pallor and sweating, leading to collapse. Absence of pulses, carotids, brachial or femorals may be noted, but this may be transitory until the dissection re-enters the lumen of the great vessel.

(9) The oesophagus

Oesophageal pain may mimic cardiac pain closely. It is usually caused by oesphageal spasm in association with hiatus hernia or reflux oesophagitis. The pain can be severe retrosternal radiating up to the throat. A history of acid reflux causing burning may be obtained and the pain may be provoked by certain hot or acidic foods, or strong alcohol and be provoked by bending or stooping or when lying flat. It is often eased by milk or alkali.

(10) Anxiety and cardiac neurosis

Chest pain is a common presenting symptom of anxiety or neurosis. Usually this pain is atypical of true cardiac pain and may be provoked by fear of heart disease or the death or affliction of a near relative or friend from heart disease. The pain is usually sharp, submammary and may be momentary or stabbing in nature or sometimes persists for days. It affects the young more commonly than the old and is not provoked by exercise nor relieved by rest. The patient shows signs of anxiety probably with other manifestations of neurosis.

Strong reassurance backed up by physical examination and a normal e.c.g. and chest X-ray will often suffice to alleviate the symptoms, or simple sedation with a small dose of diazepam is often helpful.

Summary – cardiac pain

Cardiac pain is central, retrosternal, and is not usually sharp but squeezing, vice-like, or as a weight or pressure. It is not usually in the mammary or submammary areas but most commonly radiates to the left arm or throat and less often to the right arm. If there is radiation to the arms it is down the ulnar aspects to the fingers. Unlike pain of musculo-skeletal origin, it does not persist for days but infarction pain may persist for hours and be associated with evidence of circulatory disturbance or dysrhythmias. Anginal pain has typical provocative factors and is usually relieved by rest or trinitrin. It may increase in frequency until it occurs at rest with impending infarction.

Pericardial pain is sharper in nature and is provoked or relieved by change of posture.

It should be noted that no mention has been made of *electrocardiographic changes. This is because the diagnosis of cardiac pain is essentially a clinical one in which the e.c.g. may or may not be an aid to diagnosis.* A normal e.c.g. does not exclude an infarct and the tracing may well be normal in angina but in an attack of angina, ST depression may be observed. The corollary of this is that an abnormal e.c.g. may be seen from a previous episode not related to the present attack of pain.

It is the nature and description of the pain that will lead the practitioner to diagnose it as of cardiac origin and take the appropriate action.

② Ischaemic heart disease

Myocardial ischaemia – Myocardial infarction

Myocardial ischaemia – angina pectoris

The commonest manifestation of myocardial ischaemia in practice will be angina pectoris though less commonly myocardial ischaemia may present as congestive cardiac failure. When the description of the pain is classical and the practitioner is in no doubt as to the diagnosis, he may decide on hospital referral for confirmation of the diagnosis, further investigation because the patient requests it and that it is psychologically good for the patient to be under hospital care, or that he feels uncertain of the appropriate drug therapy or diagnosis. Often the case can be managed satisfactorily by the family physician. Patients will often regard angina as a serious illness and will gain comfort and reassurance from hospital referral and assessment. Careful evaluation should be undertaken in all cases with particular reference to the following points:

(a) History,
(b) Family history,
(c) Smoking,
(d) Diet.

One must remember that concomitant conditions may cause angina, therefore:

17

Conditions associated with angina

(i) Assess the patient for anaemia, myxoedema or thyrotoxicosis.

(ii) Look for evidence of hyperlipidaemia, e.g. xanthelasma, xanthomatosis and arcus senilis.

(iii) Examine the cardiovascular system for signs of heart failure but particularly for heart murmurs. An aortic ejection systolic murmur may signify aortic stenosis which may be very relevant and more important than coronary artery disease as a cause.

(iv) Check for hypertension.

(v) Note tendency to obesity.

(vi) Observe tendency to neurosis and anxiety.

Management

In a case of angina pectoris when the decision has been taken not to refer to hospital for a consultant specialist opinion, the following *investigations* should be arranged:

Basic investigations in ischaemic heart disease

(i) Full blood picture (all types of anaemia and polycythaemia).

(ii) Fasting serum lipids (hypercholesterolaemia and lipid abnormalities).

(iii) Fasting blood sugar (diabetes mellitus).

(iv) Uric acid.

(v) Wassermann reaction (because of the remote possibility of syphilitic arteritis).

(vi) Chest X-ray (for cardiac size and evidence of pulmonary venous congestion).

(vii) An e.c.g. This should be a resting e.c.g. and should not be undertaken unless the practitioner feels proficient in interpreting the tracing when referral to hospital is indicated. If an exercise e.c.g. is required this should be performed in hospital where a DC defibrillator is available under supervision of a specialist. An *exercise e.c.g. should not be undertaken if the resting e.c.g. is abnormal.*

(viii) Thyroid function tests (myxoedema or thyrotoxicosis).

Consideration of risk factors in each patient

In the history and examination an assessment will have been made as to any risk factors that are present. These will include:

Main risk factors

(a) A family history of coronary disease or diabetes,

(b) Smoking habits of the patient,

(c) Obesity,

(d) The patients occupation i.e. whether it is stressful and particularly, whether the patient's mental state is a stressful one whether he has particular problems, business or domestic, in his life.

(e) Hypertension,

(f) The possibility of hyperlipidaemia.

If any of these are present consideration must be given to them, remembering that a patient with one risk factor is at no greater risk than his 'normal' counterpart, but thereafter risk factors are additive. Particular attention must be paid to any risk factors present and advising the patient accordingly. Notably, attacks must be made on smoking and obesity.

Treatment in relation to risk factors

Elimination of risk factors

Stress and angina

Having analysed risk factors that are present particular attention is paid to the correctable ones.

Stress is difficult to measure as a risk factor but attention should be paid to patients' psychological make-up and to stress that may be the result of domestic or occupational problems. It may be necessary to advise a patient to moderate his way of life, to discipline himself so that he has definite periods of relaxation when he should pursue other interests, sports or hobbies, or learn to delegate responsibility at work. The suggestion that the patient should change his job or occupation is usually unnecessary, unless the job is very stressful physically and undesirable in that it may well provoke more stress and anxiety. A successful, driving but tense man is not likely to take kindly to an occupation that will remove his potential success and ambition achievement and if he does so, may become resentful, frustrated and depressed. Therefore it is moderation of his life style and advice as to how he may be economical with himself and his time, allowing himself time for leisure, that is all important.

There are situations when it is necessary to recommend change of job if medical treatment has failed in treating angina, but if the patient is in this situation, it is an indication for consideration of coronary artery bypass surgery before taking this decision. Indoctrination into relaxation may be of value and sedation helpful.

Obesity and angina Many patients who are seen with *angina* and *obesity* report a marked improvement in or abolition of their symptoms after weight reduction and this initially is of greater importance than attention to lipid problems which may be corrected anyway by simple weight reduction. The symptoms of angina may totally disappear after restoration to an appropriate weight for the patient and this will be achieved by carbohydrate restriction such as:

    (i) No potatoes, rice or pasta, cakes, biscuits or puddings,

    (ii) One thin slice of bread per day,

    (iii) No added sugar,

    (iv) Restriction of alcohol,

    (v) Protein, fruit and vegetables may be taken freely.

If adhered to, this diet is usually successful and if after weight reduction an abnormal lipid pattern persists treatment may be needed by restriction of saturated fats, i.e. dairy produce (milk, butter, eggs, cream, cheese and fat meat) and the introduction of a lipid lowering agent.

Hypertension and angina Hypertension is extremely important bearing in mind the overwhelming statistical evidence of the deleterious effects of high blood pressure on morbidity and mortality mediated through the cardiovascular system. Hypertension is a key factor in the pathogenesis of coronary artery disease, though as yet there is no definite evidence that lowering blood pressure diminishes the chance of coronary thrombosis. But it has been shown to lower morbidity and mortality in cerebrovascular and renovascular disease and it is likely that this success can be extrapolated to the coronary circulation. The advent of the ß-blocking group of drugs for treatment of both angina and hypertension makes them the drugs of choice in this situation provided there are no contra-indications to their use (*vide infra*).

Hyper-lipidaemia and angina The commonest abnormal lipid patterns, Fredrickson types II and IV, are often correctable by weight reduction if the patient is overweight. If the patient is not obese a decision will be taken about drug therapy using either:

    (i) Clofibrate (Atromid S) (to be used with caution and only in clear cut cases of hypercholesterolaemia, particularly at risk.)

(ii) Cholestyramide (Questran)

(iii) Nicofuranose (Bradilan)

If the lipids are only marginally abnormal, benefit of correction is of less value than if the lipids are grossly abnormal, and dietary control by reduction of high cholesterol food intake and saturated fats may suffice. This type of dietary control is sound advice to all patients with angina and ischaemic heart disease. If a true hypercholesterolaemia of familial type is detected particularly in the presence of a bad family history of ischaemic heart disease, an energetic attack must be made to lower the cholesterol levels by giving a low cholesterol diet with a cholesterol lowering agent, clofibrate, cholestyramine or nicotinic acid, or these in combination. The detection of familial hypercholesterolaemia probably warrants referral to a cardiac or metabolic unit for full investigation and screening of the family. With increasing age and elevated cholesterol levels this group exhibits an up to ten-fold chance of coronary artery disease.

Correction of lipid abnormalities

Diabetes must be detected and treated energetically in view of the propensity of diabetic patients to develop vascular disease. Good control must be maintained by appropriate oral or insulin therapy.

Diabetes and angina

If one metabolic disorder is present others are likely and hyperuricaemia is one of them. There is evidence that it may be a factor in coronary artery disease and should be lowered by treatment with drug therapy, allopurinol (Zyloric) being the drug of choice in controlling levels, but institution of this drug may need to be covered by phenylbutazone to prevent acute gout.

Uric acid levels and angina

The deleterious effects of smoking in coronary disease are well established and the patient must be urged to cease the habit. This together with weight reduction is one of the factors that the patient can help himself with and this must be pointed out. Most success however is achieved in the post-infarct cases when the psychological shock of what has happened may cause cessation of smoking in up to 90% of post-infarct cases. A period in hospital when the habit is broken obviously aids this.

Smoking and angina

General advice

The patient should be told that most of the population have arterial narrowing from a relatively early age, some more than

21

others. There are certain factors which may accelerate the process and produce symptoms of angina. By attention to the risk factors and modification of life style, angina need not be a lifelong sentence, but only a transitory symptom or phase. Many patients have gone through a phase of it which does not recur. The patient should lose weight (if appropriate) and regulate diet to one of low saturated fats and low cholesterol, stop smoking and take exercise. This is important and bene-

Physical activity

ficial, but the form of exercise should be appropriate to the patient's age, build and previous sporting ability. In general, walking, playing golf, bicycling and swimming are good forms of exercise, but squash and other competitive sports should not be undertaken immediately though the patient may well get back to these activities with suitable retraining programmes. Sexual intercourse is an activity that the patient may hesitate to enquire about, so a positive approach should be taken on this subject pointing out that it is a normal bodily function that should be undertaken sensibly and not over-energetically, with the male assuming perhaps a rather more passive part than usual (assuming the male is the patient). Trinitrin may help prophylactically.

The patient should moderate his life style so that he has definite times of relaxation and occupations outside his work and should take proper seasonal holidays.

Drug therapy of angina
Trinitrin (glyceryl trinitrate)

GTN and TNT in angina

In simple and mild angina, drugs of the trinitrate group alone may suffice. Glyceryl trinitrate (GTN) may be used in various ways. It is usually taken sublingually with the first warning of anginal pain and allowed to dissolve. For speedier action it may be crushed in the mouth. It is also extremely effective as a prophylactic agent before an activity or situation that is known as likely to provoke angina, e.g. walking or exertion first thing on a cold morning or before a stressful meeting. The most common side-effect which may cause the patient to give up the drug is headache, severe, and often of migrainous type. This may be avoided by advising the patient to spit out the tablet as soon as anginal pain is relieved. The effect of GTN is shortlived and patients do not develop tolerance to it.

Prescribing patterns have changed noticeably in the past decade and more and more patients seen with mild angina are taking other forms of treatment, notably ß-blockers. If angina is becoming more frequent and the patient's TNT or GTN consumption is increasing, other therapy should be instituted, it may well be shown in the next few years that the incidence of myocardial infarction is less in the ß-blocked patient so that many physicians are anticipating this and using ß-blockers from the outset. TNT not only stops or prevents pain but improves cardiac performance during exercise.

ß-blockers

This group of drugs represents one of the great advances in medicine in the past fifteen years. ß-blockers are effective in ischaemic heart disease basically by lowering oxygen consumption of the myocardium and hence diminishing the likelihood of angina during exercise particularly. It can be demonstrated easily that they are effective in lessening myocardial anoxia during exercise by demonstrating the abolition of ST depression (a parameter of myocardial ischaemia) on the e.c.g. during exercise. Apart from their therapeutic effect of preventing anginal pain they have other advantages in myocardial ischaemia, notably their antidysrhythmic properties and their probable role in cardio-protection. They do however have *side-effects*, the main ones being:

Action

ß-blockers
in angina

Side-
effects

Bradycardia,
Hypotension,
Lethargy and tiredness,
Nightmares and dreams,
Raynaud's phenomenon,
Diarrhoea,
Cardiac failure,
Bronchospasm,
Muco-cutaneous syndrome.

Contra-
indications

They should *not* therefore be used in patients with bradycardia (particularly due to heart block). They may induce bradycardia which is not acceptable below a rate of 50 per minute at rest. Of the other side effects listed, ß-blockers should not be introduced in the presence of *heart failure* without full digitalization first and this needs careful consideration. In spite of the claims that the 'cardio-selective' ß-blockers do not or are less likely to cause other side effects, extreme caution must be observed in their use in *asthmatic patients* and they should only be used when the advantages and risks have been carefully weighed,

Cardio-
selective
ß-blockers

for they are capable of provoking a severe and dangerous asthmatic attack. This applies to the true asthmatic with reversible paroxysmal bronchospasm. The situation is less hazardous in the patient with chronic obstructive airways disease which is more likely associated with fixed bronchospasm. In general, true asthmatics should not be given ß-blockers unless there is an overwhelmingly strong indication to do so.

Dose levels of ß-blockers Generally, ß-blockers should be introduced at a modest dose regime in case of a marked reaction to a larger dose. Currently there are eighteen ß-blockers available in the United Kingdom, all of which are effective in their ß-blocking capacity and the choice is very much a case of individual preference and knowledge as to the dosage and manipulation of dosage regimes.

It is best to start on a relatively small dose of ß-blocker spread out in three doses per day, e.g. oxprenolol (Trasicor) 20 mg or propranolol (Inderal) 40 mg or pindolol (Visken) 5 mg t.d.s., increasing the dose subsequently. There is no doubt however that *patient compliance* is directly related to the number of doses per day and very satisfactory results may be obtained with *once or twice-daily* ß-blocker regimes.

Table 2.1 Stages in the treatment of angina

1	2	3	4	5
GTN (always) + ß-blocker (probably)	Instate or increase ß-blocker	Add nifedipine (Adalat) perhexilene (Pexid)	If no response, then consider angiography and surgery	Long-acting GTN and isosorbide

In some patients a small dose of ß-blocker may suffice, perhaps oxprenolol 20 mg b.d. and the much larger dose of slow-release oxprenolol (which may not always be slowly released) is not indicated.

Daily or twice-daily regimes Very satisfactory results have been achieved by once or twice-daily regimes using atenolol 100 mg (Tenormin), metoprolol 50–100 mg b.d., slow-release oxprenolol 160 mg (Slow Trasicor) or pindolol 15 mg (Visken). Other ß-blockers may be perfectly satisfactory but the author's preference in current practice is to maintain patients on either atenolol (Tenormin) 100 mg once daily (and this dose may be halved), metoprolol (Betaloc) 50–100 mg b.d. or slow oxprenolol 160 mg (Trasicor).

If anginal control is not achieved starting with modest

24

dose regimes, the dose of either oxprenolol (Trasicor) or propranolol (Inderal) may gradually be built up to maximal dosage levels. If this is not effective, addition of another anti-anginal drug (*vide infra*) may be helpful, or if the patient is fully ß-blocked without improvement he should probably be referred for assessment for coronary bypass surgery. A patient taking ß-blockers developing crescendo or increasingly severe and frequent angina should be admitted to hospital.

Other anti-anginal drugs

Alternatives or additions to ß-blockers

Perhexiline (Pexid) is effective but the description of unpleasant but usually reversible peripheral neuropathy has clouded the use of this drug which may still have a place. *Nifedipine* (Adalat) at a dose of 10 mg t.d.s. has proved a most *useful adjunct* to anti-anginal treatment. It is probably synergistic with the ß-blockers and can be used as a second line treatment with them but is a good alternative first line treatment in patients where ß-blockers are contra-indicated (particularly in asthmatics and bronchitics, and in heart failure and heart block).

Nifedipine works in a different way from ß-blockers, affecting calcium ion exchange across the myocardial cell membrane.

Other drugs with a place in management are long-acting GTN (Sustac) and isosorbide (Sorbitrate, Isordil). The slow-release nitrates are often effective initially but their very nature may lead to tolerance and resistance with loss of therapeutic effect. They may be of particular use, though in patients who have been shown to suffer coronary artery spasm as a cause of angina.

Diuretics may be helpful in that they improve myocardial function by diminishing myocardial work load by lowering plasma volume and hence left ventricular end diastolic pressure.

'Anti-platelet' drugs such as Anturan, clofibrate, Persantin, aspirin, all have their protagonists as a result of encouraging results, but are not yet of established value.

Coronary surgery

Results of saphenous vein bypass grafting have been impressive in their *relief* of anginal symptoms in up to 80% of patients. *Improvement* may be noted in a further 10% with an

Saphenous
vein bypass
grafting

operative mortaility not in excess of the annual mortality of anginal patients treated medically. Some authorities argue that all anginal patients should undergo coronary arteriography in the search for significant main stem coronary disease which carries a high mortality, but the logistics of this preclude its feasibility at the moment.

There is no strong evidence yet that patients operated on have a better life prognosis than those treated medically, and the main indication for referral for coronary arteriography and surgery is severe angina which has not responded to full ß-blockade and when the angina is interfering significantly with the patient's lifestyle. Coronary surgery has not yet an established place in the prevention of myocardial infarction in cases of crescendo angina, but in the next few years clarification will emerge on this point.

Main
stem
disease

Patients who have significant left coronary artery main stem disease have a better prognosis treated surgically and this diagnosis may be suspected in a patient who notices marked constitutional disturbance with anginal pain, dizziness, sweating, light headedness or syncope, and who shows marked ST depression on the exercise e.c.g. This type of patient should be referred for coronary angiography.

Myocardial infarction

When typical cardiac pain has lasted at rest for more than twenty minutes and has not been relieved by glyceryl trinitrate, the possibility must be considered that the patient is in a state of prolonged myocardial ischaemia or has had an infarction. *It is safer to assume the latter.*

Painless
infarction

Pain is usual, but in *elderly patients* infarction may be *painless* and must be considered in anyone presenting with acute *left ventricular failure* when there is no obvious underlying cause.

On many occasions, the diagnosis of myocardial infarction will be obvious, for the patient may show signs of haemodynamic disturbance with hypotension (though hypertension may initially be found), sweating, pallor, dysrhythmia and complain of feeling very unwell.

Courses of action

Procedure
after infarction

The patient may be admitted to hospital immediately from the surgery or home, or he may be sent home or kept at home

26

pending further investigations. Which of these two courses is followed will depend on the following factors:

(i) The presence of the complications of infarction.

(ii) The patient's age.

(iii) The patient's attitude to and anxiety about hospital.

(iv) The availability of a Coronary Care Unit (CCU) or Intensive Care Unit (ITU) in the near locality.

(v) The availability of domiciliary consultative services.

(vi) The availability of primary care and the doctor's own confidence and wish to look after an infarction at the home.

(vii) How long ago the infarction occurred.

Considering the above factors:

Reasons for admission to CCU

(i) If *complications* are present the patient *should be admitted to a CCU* as an emergency. The important complications are dysrhythmias (supraventricular tachycardias, ventricular extrasystoles, bradycardia or heart block), hypotension, collapse or syncope and heart failure. In all age groups the prognosis is better if such complications can be monitored in a Coronary Care Unit and dealt with quickly in a centre where all facilities are available. It is unlikely at home that the change in a patient's condition can be detected quickly enough by a relative to summon help from the family physician without putting the patient at risk. The family physician may not be skilled in dealing with these problems. Persistent pain not relieved by first line treatment may also be more effectively treated in hospital.

(ii) Age will obviously influence the decision as to whether to admit to hospital or not. Young patients or those under the age of 60 will often expect hospital admission for what to them is a potentially catastrophic event, whereas the elderly may have a fear of hospital and do as well at home assuming the infarction is uncomplicated.

<table>
<tr><td>Potential disadvantages of hospital admission</td><td>(iii)</td><td>It has frequently been suggested by various authorities that admission to hospital is emotionally so traumatic that it is likely to impede the course of the patient's illness. But myocardial infarction itself is probably more emotionally traumatic and many patients will expect admission, and will be reassured and comforted by the attention of a CCU staff and availability of equipment at a time when they rightly consider themselves very much at peril. From actual experience, it seems that patients are enormously comforted by being in a CCU and become dependent on skilled staff and often resent being moved from such a unit at the end of 48 hours or so. But here, the family physician's</td></tr>
</table>

Potential disadvantages of hospital admission

Advantages and disadvantages of CCU

(iii) It has frequently been suggested by various authorities that admission to hospital is emotionally so traumatic that it is likely to impede the course of the patient's illness. But myocardial infarction itself is probably more emotionally traumatic and many patients will expect admission, and will be reassured and comforted by the attention of a CCU staff and availability of equipment at a time when they rightly consider themselves very much at peril. From actual experience, it seems that patients are enormously comforted by being in a CCU and become dependent on skilled staff and often resent being moved from such a unit at the end of 48 hours or so. But here, the family physician's knowledge of the patient and his background is of the utmost importance in deciding this question. Apart from the patient's psychological state he will know the home, presence of children (therefore availability of rest and quiet), and the spouse's capability and attitude. There are undoubtedly a few patients who are better left at home and this is something that the family physician will assess better than a specialist on a domiciliary consultation.

(iv) There is probably no advantage in admitting an infarct patient to an hospital bed in a general ward over leaving them at home, unless home circumstances are unsuitable for rest and convalescence. Admission under the age of 65 should be to a CCU or ITU with monitoring facilities.

(v) A good, i.e. rapid, domiciliary consultative service may be of great value to the family physician in deciding on admission or not and assuming a specialist opinion can be obtained quickly at the home, this is helpful. *The patient should not be sent for an out-patient consultation or e.c.g.*

(vi) The doctor's own confidence and attitude to the problem are very important, as is the back-up which can be given on a domiciliary basis or by a primary care team.

(vii) There is little point in admitting a patient who has had an infarct two or three days before unless complications are evident. Most complications that occur are manifest in the first 48 hours so this will influence the decision.

28

Immediate action in a case of myocardial infarction

Relief of
pain

The first action must be to relieve pain and the drugs most effective in doing this also have the advantage in being anxiolytic and cause a sense of well-being. The drug of choice is diamorphine (heroin) in a dose of 5 mg given intramuscularly (or intravenously with caution). Morphine sulphate 5–10 mg or pethidine 50–100 mg are alternatives and are effective. The patient is put to rest immediately pending further action.

There may be complications evident at this early stage which should be dealt with by the general practitioner, and the common ones are:

Treatment
of
complications

(1) Left ventricular failure which should be treated by an immediate intravenous or intramuscular dose of frusemide 40 mg (Lasix).

(2) Marked bradycardia and hypotension is probably due to excessive vagal activity and can be counteracted by giving intravenous atropine 0.6 mg. The response is often dramatic. It is most likely to occur after inferior infarction and is provoked by opiate drugs.

(3) An irregular pulse may be diagnosed by auscultation of the heart or by e.c.g. as being due to ventricular extrasystoles which may herald ventricular fibrillation and should be treated with a 100 mg bolus injection of lignocaine. This drug is unlikely to prove harmful in other dysrhythmias. If the doctor has e.c.g. facilities and another dysrhythmia is evident, he may give intravenous disopyramide 10 mg (Rythmodan) which appears to be the panacea for most dysrhythmias.

Drugs which
should be
available

The following drugs therefore should be available to the general practitioner or family physician:

(i) Diamorphine, morphine or pethidine,
(ii) Atropine,
(iii) Lignocaine – intravenous 100 mg (Xylocard),
(iv) Intravenous disopyramide (Rythmodan),
(v) Intravenous frusemide 20–40 mg (Lasix).

Any drugs given in the first line situation must be documented as information to be given if hospital admission is subsequently arranged.

Subsequent action

(1) Immediate admission to hospital depending on the above criteria. This has been discussed above and need not be elaborated further here.

(2) Care of the patient at home. If the patient is to stay at home ideally a primary care nurse should spend as much time as possible with the patient with back-up and frequent visits by the family physician on subsequent days.

Treatment
in the home

General care

The patient should be put on complete bed rest for approximately the first week. This is contrary to the doctrine of some authorities who recommend early mobilization but bearing in mind that 90% of patients with infarction have significant haemodynamic disturbance due to injured myocardium, and the fact that one of the first principles of medicine is to rest an injured part, it seems prudent to rest the heart as much as possible. The patient should be allowed up for bowel action or micturition as this is often much less taxing than balancing on bed-pans, commodes or using urinal bottles.

Bed rest

Hazards of
bed rest

The patient must be told to exercise his calf muscles hourly to diminish the chance of venous thrombosis. Anticoagulation is probably safer not undertaken at home though intravenous or intramuscular heparin for 48 hours will diminish the risk of deep vein thrombosis considerably in this situation assuming there are no contra-indications to its use, such as a history of peptic ulceration or other potentially haemorrhagic gastro-intestinal lesions, hypertension or bleeding diathesis. After a week the patient begins mobilization by sitting out for half an hour in the morning and afternoon and this is gradually increased until by day four he begins to walk round his bed, bedroom, and after two weeks he is ready to descend and climb the stairs once or twice per day.

Return
to work
after
infarction

Patients who have had full infarction will need to be away from work for six to twelve weeks and by the end of the first month they are able to walk out for half a mile, be up in the house but not rising early, and resting for an hour in the afternoon. Slowly they should increase their activities aiming to be back to a normal existence by six months.

Diet after
infarction

After infarction, the diet should be light as large meals are undesirable and weight loss may be an advantage. Alcohol in moderate amounts is not contra-indicated.

Smoking and infarction

Smoking must be stopped altogether and the hazards strongly emphasized.

Drug therapy after infarction: analgesics

After the initial administration of an analgesic, a supply of a drug to relieve pain must be available to the patient. A convenient drug is tab. pethidine 50 mg taken six-hourly if necessary. Glyceryl trinitrate should also be available for use if pain recurs.

Diuretics

At the beginning of the attack if the patient is kept at home, it is advisable to administer one dose of a diuretic such as frusemide (40 mg, orally) because most patients have been found to have elevation of central venous pressure indicative of failure even if there is no clinical evidence of such. This need not be continued unless there is overt evidence of left ventricular failure.

Sedation

Simple sedation with a drug such as diazepam (Valium) is advisable. There is no proven value as yet in the use of ß-blockers routinely after infarction. Digoxin should not be used unless there is some overwhelming reason to do so, i.e. heart failure or cardiac dysrhythmia such as atrial fibrillation.

Investigations

The diagnosis of myocardial infarction should be substantiated by the following investigations:

Full blood picture and ESR

The white cell count may show a polymorph leucocytosis which may persist for up to seven days and is manifest a few hours after tissue damage has occurred. The ESR rises more slowly and may remain elevated for several weeks.

Cardiac enzymes

Elevation of enzymes

The serum glutamic oxaloacetic transaminase (SGOT) and creatinine phosphokinase (CPK) rise and fall rapidly after myocardial necrosis and usually revert to normal 72 hours after infarction. Lactic dehydrogenase (LDH) rises later and is elevated longer, being highest at three to four days and taking 14 days to return to normal.

One must remember these differences in timing, selecting, and interpreting results and also that CPK is more specific than SGOT which is present in many other tissues than the

31

heart. CPK is of course present in skeletal muscle, damage to which even by intramuscular injections can cause a rise of CPK. If enzymes are not studied in the first 48 hours, then the LDH level should be investigated because the other two enzymes will have reverted to normal.

The electrocardiograph

The basic e.c.g. changes of myocardial infarction are described in Chapter 8. The important point to remember always is that in the same way as the e.c.g. need not be confirmatory of a
Value of the e.c.g. diagnosis of angina, the e.c.g. may be normal in the early stages of infarction and the diagnosis is essentially a clinical one on which subsequent action is based.

An e.c.g. should be performed however to aid diagnosis or to document it. The latter is important as a wrong diagnosis may label a patient with a serious condition which he has not got, with the ensuing problems of life insurance, job promotion and the patient's anxiety.

The e.c.g. will be performed either at the patient's home, by the family physician or a consultant, at the surgery or in hospital. If it is normal it should be repeated 24 or 48 hours later as it may take this time for the characteristic changes to appear. The patient with suspected infarction must not be sent to hospital for an out-patient e.c.g.

General considerations

Uncertain diagnosis If the diagnosis of infarction is *uncertain*, it is sensible to *admit* the patient to a *CCU* or *ITU* where serial e.c.gs may be performed and interpreted along with serial cardiac enzyme changes, and most hospitals will accept patients on this basis and will discharge the patient quickly if infarction is excluded.

When the diagnosis has been confirmed, the general practitioner will be looking after the patient at home through the acute phase and convalescence or will take over the case on the patient's discharge from hospital.
General management In either situation it is important to adopt an attitude of optimism pointing out that the patient should be able to lead a normal life again after three to six months, that infarction can be a 'cure' for both angina and hypertension if these conditions pre-existed.

The doctor must consider the risk factors of coronary artery disease and determine which ones are present in the patient and give the relevant advice, with particular accent on weight loss and smoking.

Patient's life style

It is usually not necessary to advise a change of job, as doing so will create many problems in the life of a patient and promote more anxiety. Moderation of life style and work-style is very different and these may well need alteration and advice. It is as well to remember that a man or woman will do their own job which they know well, even if it is a manual and physical job, more easily and efficiently than something that is new. A manual worker may often be able to delegate the hard physical work in the months after infarction. Similarly an office worker may, with the co-operation of his employer, be able to resume work initially at reduced hours.

Type of work

Hours of work

Interests and hobbies

The patient should be encouraged to increase slowly his exercise or take up outside interests in hobbies or sport of a non-competitive nature. There is no good evidence that programmed gymnasium activities are particularly beneficial.

Sexual intercourse

Sexual intercourse may be resumed, an anxiety and doubt uppermost in the minds of many patients, but should be practised sensibly and not over-energetically, but if anginal pain is provoked, glyceryl trinitrate may be used prophylactically, as it may before any other form of exertion likely to promote pain.

The co-operation of the patient's spouse must be sought in all these matters and he or she should be given a full explanation of the events that have occurred and what the programme for the future is.

Sport

Gradual resumption of physical activities will be followed in the three to six months period after an uncomplicated infarction. Such activities as swimming, walking and bicycling are to be encouraged. Patients who have been physically inactive prior to infarction should be encouraged to alter their style of life but should do this with moderation. It would not be suitable for a middle-aged man previously unathletic to start playing squash or hard tennis or competitive sport. Common sense and moderation are necessary and a post-infarction patient must not become fanatical about exercise and sporting activity.

③ Hypertension

Presentation – General considerations – Investigations – The treatment of hypertension – Notes on hypotensive drugs

Presentation

Chance or routine finding
Cardiomegaly on routine chest X-ray
Headache
Epistaxis
Ophthalmic examination
Renal failure
Left ventricular or congestive failure
Pregnancy
Cerebro vascular accident

General considerations

Defining hypertension It is extremely difficult to define hypertension other than to state that it is high systemic arterial pressure, for such a definition must always take into account age. It is the blood pressure in the light of the age that will determine whether to treat or not, for a man of 65 with a pressure of 160/100 is a very different proposition to a man of 25 with the same pressure.

The treatment of blood pressure has improved considerably since the advent of the ß-blocking drugs; before their introduction most hypotensive agents caused side effects which were often unacceptable. There is as yet no perfect hypotensive agent, i.e. one that is effective and is totally free of

35

side-effects, though the ß-blockers have gone a long way toward this goal.

In deciding to treat a patient, the balance of advantages of reduced morbidity and mortality against disadvantages of treatment must be considered. The advantages of treating hypertension in reducing its deleterious effects on the cerebro-vascular and renal arterial circulation are well established and there is optimism that prospective trials will show the same advantages on the coronary artery circulation. But long-term therapy is a constant reminder to patients that they have a potential circulatory problem and even the ß-blockers have some side effects. The patient's age and height of pressure are the important factors here and it must be emphasized that an elevated systolic pressure is as harmful as an elevated diastolic pressure, as is evident from the results of the Framingham studies.

But the results of treatment are clear and unequivocal. If the blood pressure is lowered, morbidity and mortality are significantly lowered.

Causes of hypertension

(1) Essential or primary

(2) Renal – arterial disease
parenchymal disease

(3) Coarctation of aorta

(4) Endocrine – Cushing's syndrome
phaeochromocytoma
Conn's tumour
acromegaly
pregnancy
hypercalcaemia

(5) Oral contraception

History

Hypertension is usually asymptomatic and a chance finding. It may be a cause of headache or epistaxis. It is important to try to establish the duration of high blood pressure by asking if the patient has had it recorded before at routine medical examination, for life insurance, service entry or during pregnancy.

The patient may volunteer symptoms related to hypertension but if not, the presence of angina pectoris, peripheral vascular disease or heart failure must be sought by appropriate questioning.

Family history The presence of hypertension in the family history must be found, as must premature deaths in the family from vascular disease and hypertension be tactfully sought.

Symptoms suggestive of renal cause Perhaps the most important aspect of the patient's history is to enquire of any symptoms related to urinary tract infections in the past or present, such as dysuria or frequency which may give a clue to a renal anomaly or more particularly, chronic or recurrent pyelonephritis.

The contraceptive pill Further questioning should determine whether females have been hypertensive in pregnancy, have had toxaemia of pregnancy or whether they are or have been taking the contraceptive pill.

Patient's disposition An assessment of the patient's psychological state must be made by enquiring into anxiety, stress at work or at home, and an assessment made from these as to his attitude to life, whether he is a worrier who experiences periods of stress which in the younger groups may give rise to paroxysmal systolic hypertension.

Examination

Recording the blood pressure The blood pressure should be recorded with the patient lying and standing and should be repeated after resting for five minutes reclining. The systolic phase should be recorded together with the fifth phase representing the diastolic figure.

Examination of CVS The cardiovascular system is examined, noting particularly evidence of left ventricular hypertrophy by palpation, and added third or fourth heart sounds by auscultation. The femoral pulses must be palpated for absence or delay suggestive of coarctation of the aorta. The abdomen should be

Fundoscopy auscultated for renal artery bruits (renal artery stenosis), and the fundi examined for evidence of hypertensive retinopathy.

Endocrine abnormalities Evidence of endocrine abnormalities should be looked for, e.g. the features of Cushing's syndrome or acromegaly.

Investigations
General
Chest X-ray

This is mainly to determine heart size and left ventricular hypertrophy and the presence of pulmonary venous congestion.

37

The electrocardiogram

This is recorded to assess left ventricular hypertrophy and strain pattern. The presence of either will accentuate the need for treatment.

Renal investigations
Mid-stream urine (MSU)

Searching for a renal cause
The one vital investigation in general practice is to diagnose the presence of renal infection and preferrably two MSU specimens should be taken. If infection is overlooked, hypertension may accelerate and provoke renal failure. With this in mind, the MSU must be analysed for blood and protein and by microscopy for the presence of pus cells and organisms, the latter being confirmed by bacteriological culture.

Blood urea and creatinine levels

If either of these are abnormal, it is advisable to assess renal function more accurately by a creatinine clearance test.

Intravenous pyelogram (IVP)

This examination should be performed on any hypertensive patient under the age of 50 years, its particular value being the exclusion of unilateral renal disease. If unilateral renal disease is seen, the patient should be referred to a specialist unit for further investigation. Some causes of unilateral renal disease, e.g. renal artery stenosis or hydronephrosis, may be amenable to surgery in a case of hypertension. The presence of chronic pyelonephritis may be suggested from the IVP which will justify further investigation and possibly affect treatment.

Radioactive renogram

Access to this test may not be possible through general practice but it is an extremely useful and easy test to exclude unilateral renal disease.

Endocrine investigations

It is unlikely and probably unnecessary that these will be undertaken routinely unless there is a hint from examination and history that there is an endocrine anomaly present.

,Electrolytes and urea

Electrolytes and Conn's tumour

A low serum potassium level may give a clue to the presence of a Conn's tumour and would justify referral for further investigation. A low serum potassium is found however in a proportion of hypertensive subjects.

An elevated sodium level and low potassium may be seen in Cushing's syndrome.

Phaeochromocytoma

Catechol-amines

In a patient who shows a marked paroxysmal rise in blood pressure often associated with sweating, pallor, tachycardia and headache, 24 hour urine collections should be assayed for the breakdown products of catecholamines (VMA). The urine should be collected in a suitable container with additive and certain foods and drugs withheld. (Details of these should be ascertained from the biochemical laboratory.)

Blood calcium level

Preferably fasting blood taken from an uncuffed arm vein.

Steroid levels

An elevated random cortisol may give support to the clinical impression of Cushing's syndrome in which event one should proceed to perform a test to show loss of diurnal variation of steroid secretion and then perform a dexamethasone suppression test.

The decision to treat hypertension

The decision to treat or not will have been taken in the light of the patient's age and the height of systolic and diastolic pressures, remembering that the systolic level is as important as the diastolic. Very definite indications to treat hypertension are:

Clear indications to ᾽ treat

(i) When there is evidence of left ventricular strain on e.c.g.

(ii) If there is incipient or overt left ventricular failure.

(iii) If the fundi show hypertensive retinopathy.

(iv) *If there is evidence of renal impairment.* Even gross

renal impairment may be reversed if satisfactory blood pressure control is obtained but this must be done under careful monitoring of renal function by serum creatinine and urea levels.

(v) After cerebrovascular accidents.

Grades of hypertension

Three groups of hypertensive patients are described, mild, moderate and severe. The mild cases often have paroxysmal systolic hypertension related to stress and are in the younger age group. Such patients are detected at routine medical examinations. There is evidence to suggest that they may become 'fixed' hypertensives later. The decision to treat this group is not easy. Below the age of 45 patients with a diastolic pressure of 95 mmHg or over and systolic levels of 145 mmHg or above warrant treatment in the author's view, or if not treated, follow-up is mandatory. Some latitude may be allowed for women, who tolerate high pressure better in the lower age groups.

Severe hypertension

Severe hypertension, that is 190 mmHg systolic or above, 115 mmHg diastolic or above, will always warrant treatment. The only possible exception is in the elderly for there is no positive evidence that treating high pressure over the age of 70 is beneficial but it is probably advisable to lower systolic levels of 180 or more in the elderly. It is probably inadvisable to lower pressure too much in the older age group for fear of diminished cerebral and coronary perfusion. When measuring blood pressure in the elderly one is uncertain if the pressure represents truly the intraluminal pressure, or that pressure necessary to compress an arteriosclerotic vessel.

Significance of blood pressure in the elderly

Moderate hypertension, where the systolic pressure is 150–190 mmHg, and the diastolic value 95–120 mmHg, will usually justify treatment but age must be taken into account. In any of these groups, the decision to treat will be reinforced by the presence of any vascular impairment in the heart, kidneys or eyes.

Aims of treatment and pressure levels

Level of improvement of pressure

It is unusual and inadvisable to aim to restore severe hypertension to normal figures for the patient's age. This could make the patient feel very unwell and can lead to renal, coronary or cerebrovascular insufficiency. It is the percentage improvement that matters and an initial pressure of, for example, 230/130 may be reduced to 170/110 and be acceptable. The patient is at considerably less risk. In mild hypertension, a normal figure is often restored by modest doses of drugs.

The aim of treatment is that by reducing pressure, systolic or diastolic, the morbidity and mortality risks are similarly reduced without making the patient's life intolerable from side effects.

The treatment of hypertension

In all grades of hypertension, mild, moderate and severe, treatment with the ß-blockers, is the treatment of choice assuming the patient is not asthmatic, is not in heart failure and has not got heart block.

Groups of drugs used in hypertension

Choice of drugs

(1) Simple sedation (diazepam)
(2) Diuretics (Navidrex-K, Hygroton, Moduretic)
(3) ß-blockers (oxprenolol, atenolol, pindolol)
(4) 'Vascular' drugs (hydralazine, prazosin)
(5) Others – methyl dopa
        clonidine
        guanethidine
        debrisoquine
        indapamide
        minoxidil (Loniten)

Suggested regime of hypotensive drugs

(1) ß-blockers,
    (if ß-blockers are contra-indicated start at (2)),
(2) add diuretics,
(3) add hydralazine (Hydergine),
    or prazosin (Hypovase),
(4) Indapamide (Natrilix),
    or clonidine (Catapres),
(5) Methyl dopa (Aldomet),
    guanethidine (Ismelin),
    bethanidine (Esbatal),
    debrisoquine (Declinax).
(6) Consiaer minoxidil if severe and persistent hypertension.

Mild hypertension

Anxiety and hypertension

If anxiety plays a part, simple sedation with a drug such as diazepam (Valium) may be beneficial but as most ß-blockers are in part anxiolytic they are preferable. A mild paroxysmal

Paroxysmal
hypertension

hypertensive patient will often respond well to a small twice or even once daily dose of a ß-blocker, e.g. oxprenolol (Trasicor) 20 mg b.d. or pindolol (Visken) 5 mg b.d. An alternative is a once daily dose of atenolol (Tenormin) 50–100 mg daily, but in this group the slow-release preparation of ß-blockers may give too large a dose of ß-blocker too quickly.

If control on a small dose is not achieved, the dose may be increased, a diuretic added and this will usually suffice. For convenience and patient compliance the ß-blocker may be converted to a slow-release once daily regime.

Moderate and severe hypertension

Higher doses
of ß-blockers

ß-blockers in larger doses should be instated. Atenolol 100 mg daily, doubling this dose if required, or oxprenolol 40 mg t.d.s. or propranolol 20 mg t.d.s. together with a diuretic such as cyclopenthiazide (Navidrex-K) ii o.m. are all suitable regimes. If control is not achieved, the ß-blocker may be increased to maximum dosage. If this is not successful the current practice is to add a drug such as hydralazine (starting dose 25 mg t.d.s.) or prazosin (1 mg t.d.s.), for these drugs work synergistically with ß-blockers. If control is still not achieved, a different hypotensive agent such as guanethidine or bethanidine should be added. If control is not satisfactory it is advisable to refer the patient for a specialist opinion about treatment (see regime of treatment).

In extreme and severe persistent hypertension, the peripheral vasodilator minoxidil (Loniten) may be used. This drug is limited to hospital practice because of its side effect of hirsutism.

Treatment in special groups
Pregnancy

Problems
in special
groups

ß-blockers are not used routinely having not been proven as being non-teratogenic, though they probably are so but they cause fetal bradycardia which makes detection of fetal distress difficult. Methyl dopa (Aldomet) is the drug of choice, starting at a dose of 250 mg t.d.s. A diuretic may need to be added.

Asthmatics

ß-blockers should not be used unless there is an overwhelming reason to do so. One of the second line drugs with a diuretic is advised. Prazosin is preferred being less likely to cause a tachycardia without a ß-blocker than hydralazine.

Heart failure

ß-blockers should not be given until the patient is digitalized and taking a diuretic. If urgent control is needed intramuscular hydralazine is the best drug before failure is controlled.

Hypertensive crisis or accelerated hypertension

Intramuscular or intravenous hydralazine is the safest drug to administer to control severe hypertension as in the accelerated phase of hypertension. Patients with *hypertensive crisis* or with the *accelerated phase* of hypertension justify *immediate hospital admission.*

Notes on hypotensive drugs
ß-blockers

Summarizing the hypotensive drugs

Relatively free of side effects, they are the first line drugs in treatment of hypertension and the mainstay (see Chapter 12). In many cases they are sufficient to control pressure alone.

Diuretics

Diuretics may be sufficient in mild hypertension alone, but are best used in conjunction with ß-blockers. In mild and moderate cases, ß-blockers lower systolic pressure and the addition of a diuretic seems to lower diastolic levels.

Short acting diuretics should not be used in treatment of hypertension. The long acting thiazides are the best, e.g. cyclopenthiazide, bendrofluazide (Navidrex-K, Neo-Naclex-K). Frusemide and bumetanide are not indicated. Diuretics alone may be used in elderly hypertensives.

Vascular acting drugs

Hydralazine and prazosin are used. The former drug, out of favour for some years because of lupus erythematosus phenomenon is safe in doses below 200 mg daily. Like prazosin (which may have more subjective side-effects) this drug is synergistic with ß-blockers. There are encouraging early reports of a newly released α-blocker, indoramin (Baratol) which may prove an important addition to this group.

Other drugs

Methyl dopa – for a time the mainstay of treatment, this drug causes marked subjective side effects e.g. lethargy, tiredness, depression, failure to ejaculate, haemolytic anaemia. It is no longer a first line drug. Guanethidine, debrisoquine, and bethanidine are post-ganglionic blockers and these drugs may cause postural hypotension, bowel disturbance, and impotence. No longer a first choice, they may be added to first line regimes. Clonidine (Catapres) is of value as a fourth line drug but causes depression and a dry mouth. Also it may cause rebound hypertension on cessation. Certainly it is of value when hypertension is associated with migrainous headache.

Indapamide (Natrilix) is a new drug taken in once daily dose and reported so far to be free of side effects. It may have an important place as an alternative to ß-blockers, and can be added to ß-blockers or used when ß-blockers are contra-indicated.

Minoxidil (Loniten) may be used in severe hypertension not controlled by the other drugs. It is potent and effective as a peripheral vasodilator and lowers peripheral resistance. However, as it may cause marked new or increased hair growth on the face, back arms shoulders or legs its treatment will only be instituted by a specialist unit. It is given in twice daily dosage starting at 10 mg increasing to a maximum 100 mg daily.

Indoramin (Baratol) is new but could become an alternative first choice in patients who cannot take ß-blockers. At the moment its value would seem to be as a good alternative vascular acting drug to prazosin or hydralazine. Hydralazine is very suitable with a ß-blocker but alone may cause unacceptable tachycardia.

Cardiac murmurs

Systolic murmurs – Diastolic murmurs

Detection of murmurs

Cardiac murmurs will be noticed at routine medical examinations, e.g. for life insurance, when patients are examined for other reasons and complaints, and when patients present with symptoms of heart disease such as breathlessness due to heart failure, and angina. If murmurs are associated with symptoms, further investigations and a specialist opinion will be necessary. It is essential to determine whether murmurs are significant and organic in origin, or are innocent and of no significance. The loudness of a murmur does not correlate with degree of organic disease. Murmurs must not be ignored but must be diagnosed by the family physician or after specialist referral.

Types of murmur

In this chapter, no attempt is made to describe the diagnosis of complicated heart defects as in severe congenital heart disease, only to give an aid in determining the significance of murmurs that are likely to be heard in day to day practice.

Murmurs are either systolic or diastolic. Systolic murmurs may be of *organic significance*, diastolic murmurs are *always* so.

Timing a murmur

The timing of a murmur should be determined by auscultation of the heart at the point of maximal intensity of the murmur, and by palpating a carotid vessel and timing the murmur against the systolic pulse wave felt. If it is synchronous

45

with the pulse wave it is systolic, otherwise it is diastolic.

Having determined if a murmur is systolic or diastolic, its intensity, timbre and relationship to the heart sounds are noted. After this, the key areas of auscultation are listened to, to determine propagation of a murmur, and the presence of other murmurs.

Systolic murmurs

Types of systolic murmur

Systolic murmurs are commonly of two types, either *pan-systolic* which means that the murmur extends from the first to the second heart sounds and are of the same intensity throughout:

Pan-systolic

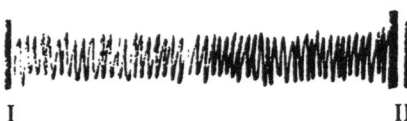

I   II

or ejection systolic, when both heart sounds can be heard distinct from the murmur which has mid-systolic accentuation:

Ejection systolic

I   II

Pan-systolic murmurs – causes

All of these causes may be congenital or acquired, and include:

Mitral regurgitation (MR)
Ventricular septal defect (VSD)
Tricuspid regurgitation (TR)

The *commonest cause* of a pan-systolic murmur is *mitral regurgitation*. This murmur is heard maximally in the mitral area and is propagated laterally to the left axilla. It may also be heard at the left sternal edge but it is heard maximally at the apex and out to the axilla. The murmur is blowing in quality.

The murmur of a ventricular septal defect is also pan-systolic in timing, but this murmur is heard maximally at the left sternal edge over the fourth or fifth intercostal space. Its intensity becomes less towards the apex and it is usually harsh in quality.

Tricuspid regurgitation produces a blowing pan-systolic murmur over the lower end of the sternum. It may be heard toward the apex and the murmur is accentuated by deep inspiration due to increased venous filling of the right side of the heart. (Other features of tricuspid regurgitation are marked systolic venous waves (V waves) in the neck and hepatic pulsation.)

Differentiation of pan-systolic murmurs

Mitral regurgitation

Mitral regurgitation is usually of rheumatic origin and may be associated with other valvular lesions which will support the diagnosis. The chest X-ray may show enlargement of the left atrium, sometimes very marked, left ventricular enlargement and pulmonary venous congestion. The electrocardiograph may show atrial fibrillation (supportive evidence of a rheumatic aetiology) left ventricular hypertrophy and strain.

Tricuspid regurgitation

The murmur of tricuspid regurgitation is unusually heard alone because there are likely to be other valves involved. But tricuspid regurgitation usually produces very classical signs apart from the murmur, notably large systolic waves in the jugular veins (V waves) and a pulsatile liver. The chest X-ray may show right atrial enlargement and the e.c.g. may indicate right atrial strain.

Ventricular septal defect

The murmur of a *VSD* may not be associated with any other signs for if the defect is *small* the murmur is loud and associated with a thrill *(maladie de Roger)*. This murmur is more likely to be heard in children and the murmurs eventually disappear with growth as the defect closes. Electrocardiogram and chest X-ray are likely to be normal.

A *large VSD* may be associated with symptoms due to significant left to right shunting and the *chest X-ray* is likely to show pleonaemia of the lung fields, *left atrial enlargement* and biventricular enlargement or pulmonary hypertension. The e.c.g. may show right and left ventricular hypertrophy and pulmonary hypertension.

Cardiac dilatation and pan-systolic murmurs

Dilated mitral valve Various conditions that cause significant heart enlargement may cause dilatation of the mitral ring and hence mitral regurgitation. Thus this type of murmur may appear in many cases of heart failure and is usually pan-systolic. Similarly, in severe failure leading to pulmonary hypertension, the pan-systolic murmur of tricuspid regurgitation may appear to disappear temporarily after treatment.

Late systolic murmurs

Posterior cusp prolapse Late systolic murmurs heard at the apex at any stage may signify a posterior cusp prolapse causing mitral regurgitation; this is clinically not significant, until later in life.

Late systolic murmur

I   II

Ejection systolic murmurs

The various causes of ejection systolic murmurs are:

(1) Aortic area

Aortic stenosis

Causes of ejection murmurs Congenital: valvar
supravalvar
subvalvar

Acquired: rheumatic
idiopathic acquired
calcific
(elderly)

Aortic sclerosis: arteriosclerosis

(2) Pulmonary area
Pulmonary stenosis

Congenital: valvar
infundibular

Acquired: rheumatic (rare)

48

Atrial septal defect

Innocent or pulmonary flow murmur

Aortic area ejection murmurs

The murmur and features of aortic stenosis

In cases of aortic stenosis the murmur is harsh or grunting in quality and is propagated upwards from the aortic area into the neck and is heard over the carotid arteries. This may be associated with a small, slow rising pulse due to low pulse pressure unless the defect is subvalvar when the pulse is 'bouncy'. The chest X-ray will show left ventricular hypertrophy and enlargement, and the e.c.g. will show left ventricular strain.

Aortic sclerosis

Aortic sclerosis

Aortic sclerosis produces a murmur commonly heard in the elderly and of little haemodynamic significance. The murmur is caused by flow across a roughened sclerosed valve. The murmur is like that of aortic stenosis but is associated with a normal pulse pressure, normal chest X-ray and no left ventricular strain pattern on the e.c.g.

Pulmonary area ejection murmurs

Murmur and features of pulmonary stenosis

In cases of pulmonary stenosis, the systolic murmur may be associated with an ejection click if the lesion is valvar. The second heart sound is likely to be single.

The chest X-ray will show oligaemia of the lung fields and perhaps a post-valvar stenotic dilatation. The e.c.g. may show right ventricular preponderance or strain.

Atrial septal defect

Where there is an atrial septal defect, it is usually possible to hear the ejection systolic murmur in association with fixed splitting of the second heart sound, i.e. the aortic and pulmonary components do not move with respiration as they do normally. Chest X-ray may show overfilling of the lung fields with blood and the e.c.g. a right bundle branch pattern.

Innocent murmur

In many states which cause an increased circulatory rate, an ejection murmur is heard in the pulmonary area as blood flows through the pulmonary valve in systole. This is likely to be an innocent or pulmonary flow murmur.

Such a murmur is heard in the young, in pregnancy, in febrile children and idiopathically in the young. It is unassociated with any haemodynamic disturbance, so the e.c.g. and chest X-ray appear normal and the patient is asymptomatic. The second heart sound 'splits' and 'moves' normally. This murmur is the one most commonly heard in the surgery, office or consulting room, and is a common cause of referral. If mis-diagnosed, it will result in unnecessary anxiety and penalties. The murmur is likely to disappear with time, growth and change of haemodynamic state. If doubt exists about its significance the patient should be seen occasionally over years for review of the murmur, the chest X-ray and e.c.g. but all the time the patient must be reassured.

Conclusion

The cause of pulmonary area ejection murmurs is usually to be determined by:

Key factors in determining the significance of a pulmonary ejection murmur

(i) Careful auscultation of the *second sound* to determine whether it is *single* (pulmonary stenosis) *widely* or *fixedly* split (ASD).

(ii) Looking at the e.c.g. – right bundle branch block (ASD), right ventricular strain (pulmonary stenosis).

(iii) Examining the chest X-ray for oligaemia (pulmonary stenosis) and pleonaemia (ASD).

If these are *all normal* and the patient asymptomatic, the murmur is likely to be an *innocent one*.

Diastolic murmurs

These are always organic and significant. There are two types – mid-diastolic and early diastolic.

Different timing of diastolic murmurs

Mid-diastolic murmurs are usually low pitched or rumbling. They commence in mid-diastole and may be short or long. They may accentuate before the first heart sound.

Mid-diastolic murmurs

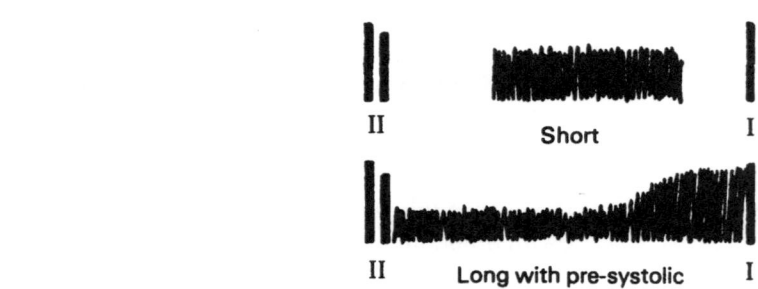

I   II   Short   I

I   II   Long with pre-systolic accentuation   I

Cardiac murmurs

Early diastolic murmurs are usually soft or blowing, and they may be very quiet almost like a soft breath sound.

Early
diastolic
murmur

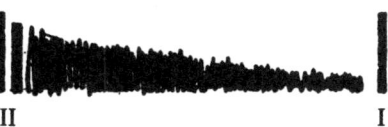

I   II   I

Diastolic murmurs in mitral area

Causes of
diastolic
murmurs in
mitral area

The cause of diastolic murmurs in the mitral area are:

Mitral stenosis: Congenital
                      Acquired
                      Rheumatic
                      Calcific of the elderly

Tricuspid stenosis: Congenital
                        Rheumatic

Aortic regurgitation (*mid-diastolic* murmur of *Austin Flint*).

Mitral stenosis

The murmur
of mitral
stenosis

The murmur is heard most easily at the apex or just lateral to it. Accentuation of the murmur is produced by listening to the heart with the patient in the left lateral position. The murmur is a low-pitched rumbling or vibratory noise of very characteristic note. In association with it, one is likely to hear a loud first sound and an opening snap, a sharp short sound just after the second sound. If the patient is in sinus rhythm the murmur will have pre-systolic crescendo due to the rapid increase of blood flow across the mitral valve with the late atrial systolic contraction.

Chest
X-ray
Electro-
cardiogram

Chest X-ray may show slight left atrial enlargement, congestion of the lung fields and possibly Kerly's B lines. If in sinus rhythm, the P waves on the e.c.g. may show P mitrale, a bifid broad P wave produced by left atrial strain.

Tricuspid stenosis

Features of
tricuspid
stenosis

This murmur is very similar in quality to that of mitral stenosis but is usually heard more medially, starting over the lower sternal area and spreading laterally to the mitral area. It is likely to be in association with other valve lesions. The venous pulse in the neck shows a slow descent of the venous pulse as blood flow meets tricuspid obstruction.

The chest X-ray will probably show right atrial enlargement and the e.c.g. right atrial strain with a peaked P wave.

The mid-diastolic murmur (Austin Flint)

Austin Flint mid-diastolic murmurs This short mid-diastolic murmur is heard at the apex and may be confused with the murmur of mild mitral stenosis. It is due to the jet of blood from an incompetent and regurgitant aortic valve striking the anterior leaflet of the mitral valve causing it to reverberate.

Unless mitral stenosis is actually present, other clinical features of mitral stenosis are not evident but careful auscultation should show the presence of an aortic regurgitant (i.e. early diastolic) murmur.

Diastolic murmurs in aortic area

Causes of aortic diastolic murmurs

Causes:	Congenital
	Marfans syndrome
Acquired:	Rheumatic
	Endocarditis
	Ankylosing spondylitis
	Syphilis
	Trauma

The murmur of aortic regurgitation occurs at the very onset of diastole, is often very soft and blowing in quality and is probably the most difficult of all cardiac murmurs to hear. Its detection is aided by sitting the patient forward and listening carefully during held expiration. The murmur may, in fact, be heard more easily down the left sternal border or even at the lower end of the sternum, which is sometimes the only place it may be heard.

Features of aortic regurgitation If the lesion is insignificant, there may be no other signs present but if it is severe, the diastolic pressure is found to be low giving rise to a wide pulse pressure, the collapsing type of pulse with marked arterial pulsation in the neck (Corrigan's sign).

Left ventricular enlargement is seen on chest X-ray and the e.c.g. will show left ventricular strain.

Cardiac murmurs

Diastolic murmur in the pulmonary area

The causes of these murmurs are:

Pulmonary incompetence: Congenital
                        Acquired
                        Rheumatic or secondary to
                        pulmonary hypertension

Patent ductus arteriosus

Pulmonary incompetence

This murmur is early in timing, is soft and very like that of
aortic regurgitation without the 'bouncy' or 'collapsing' type of
arterial pulse. It is often secondary to pulmonary hypertension
of which there will be other evidence such as right ventricular
hypertrophy and a loud pulmonary second sound.

Patent ductus arteriosus

This diastolic murmur will be heard in the pulmonary area in
association with a systolic murmur producing a continuous
murmur through systole and diastole, the so-called machinery
murmur. It may be difficult to differentiate it from the to-and-
fro murmur (systolic and diastolic murmur) of mixed aortic
stenosis and regurgitation. On chest X-ray the aortic arch is
small and the lungs overfilled with blood unless the shunt has
reversed.

Combined systolic and diastolic murmurs

Combined
systolic and
diastolic
murmurs

Mixed valve
lesions

The presence of a combined systolic and diastolic murmur
means that a mixed valve lesion is present and the qualities
and features that have been described above will pertain to
both. This situation is common, and experience will enable the
practitioner to diagnose, for example, mixed mitral stenosis
and regurgitation in the presence of aortic regurgitation but
this problem is more relevant to cardiology as a specialty and
not to the interpretation of murmurs as heard in a clinic,
surgery or office. No attempt will be made here to resolve the
problem as to which is the predominant and significant lesion.
Reference to a more detailed cardiological textbook is necessary.

Summary

Cardiac murmurs are heard commonly. Many are of innocent significance but simple steps with e.c.g.s and chest X-rays, together with the search for other signs, will determine those of organic significance.

Diastolic murmurs are always of organic significance.

5 Syncope

Dysrhythmias – Valvular heart disease – Congenital heart disease – Hypotension – Other low output states – Pulmonary embolism – Cardiac compression

Presentation

Episodes of impaired consciousness either complete or incomplete are common presenting symptoms at a doctor's surgery. The greatest problem and need is to determine whether these attacks are epileptic in nature or whether they are syncopal. The patient often complains of 'queer turns'.

In this chapter, the cardiac causes of syncope are to be considered though it must be remembered that a cardiac problem that causes a fall in cardiac output may provoke true epilepsy in a patient who has an epileptic tendency or an epileptogenic focus in the brain.

The nature of syncope
In a patient with true syncope, that is loss or impairment of consciousness for a few seconds, usually, though not always, occurring in a sitting or standing position, cardiac causes must be borne in mind. Similarly the very common symptom of 'I keep coming over queer doctor', may have a cardiac cause and studies using continuous monitoring systems in these groups of patients have shown that up to 20% of them may have cardiac dysrhythmias.

Any defect that results in diminished perfusion of brain tissue may cause impairment of the conscious level.

Cardiac causes of syncope
The defects that are met commonly in practice are due to:

(1) Dysrhythmias of the heart,
(2) Valvular heart disease,

55

(3) Congenital heart disease,
(4) Hypotension,
(5) Other low output states,
(6) Pulmonary embolism,
(7) Cardiac compression.

Dysrhythmias

Any disorder of the heart beat which results in alteration of the normally efficient sinus rhythm to a less efficient one may cause a *fall* of *stroke volume* and hence cardiac output and cerebral perfusion. Patients who give a classical description of paroxysmal tachycardia often describe the symptoms of faintness, feeling unreal or lightheaded during the attack.

Paroxysmal supraventricular tachycardia

Paroxysmal tachycardia as a cause of syncope

In this situation, the patient describes rapid regular heart beats in the attacks, which may occur at all ages and are certainly not uncommon in the young with healthy hearts. This is probably the commonest type of dysrhythmia encountered in practice and may be provoked by anxiety, fear, bending or stooping, large meals or excesses of alcohol or smoking. The attack may last for seconds or many hours but is usually

Treatment

tolerated well. The attack may be terminated by vagal stimulation with carotid massage, pressure on the eye balls, the Valsalva manoeuvre or drinking ice water. If the attack persists, antidysrhythmic drugs such as disopyramide (Rythmodan), intravenous practolol (Eraldin) or verapamil (Cordilox) may be necessary but if these fail and the attack persists for several hours, DC cardioversion is indicated. These measures should be undertaken in hospital under e.c.g. monitoring control, and certainly warrant a specialist's opinion. Such drugs should not be administered outside hospital.

Prophylaxis

Simple sedation may be helpful as a prophylactic measure, or antidysrhythmic drugs indicated if attacks are frequent and troublesome.

Paroxysmal atrial fibrillation and flutter

Intermittent atrial fibrillation and flutter

Paroxysmal fibrillators often convert from a normal sinus rhythm to a very rapid fibrillation or flutter. This results in a very poor stroke volume and cardiac output with resultant impairment of the conscious level.

Further, dysrhythmias of this type may lead to left atrial thrombus formation with resultant *embolism to the brain* which can give rise to transient ischaemic attacks. This is more likely to occur in association with mitral valve disease. There are many causes of paroxysmal fibrillation and flutter and organic heart disease as a cause is more likely than in the paroxysmal supraventricular tachycardia group. Underlying conditions such as thyrotoxicosis, ischaemic heart disease, rheumatic heart disease, cardiomyopathy, drugs and alcohol are considered, though in a large group there is no detectable cause, the so-called *'lone fibrillators'*. An attack may need to be terminated in hospital by antidysrhythmic drugs or DC cardioversion.

Prophylactic drug therapy may be necessary and success obtained by the use of *long-acting quinidine* preparations (Kinidin Durules), or the actual cardiac rate controlled in an attack by the use of digitalis.

There are favourable reports with amiodarone (Cordarone X) in treating paroxysmal atrial fibrillation and other supraventricular tachycardias.

Underlying causes (margin)

Prophylaxis (margin)

Ventricular tachycardias

When the ventricle takes on its own rhythm, *ventricular tachycardias* are much more likely to result in impairment of consciousness than supraventricular ones because the rhythm is very much less efficient and results in an extremely *low output state*. Ventricular fibrillation or flutter is not as uncommon as one might imagine as 24 hour e.c.g. tape monitoring studies have shown even in persons with no other cardiac symptoms.

If they persist, they are tolerated far less well than supraventricular tachycardias and are much more likely to provoke cardiac pain and failure. They may herald cardiac arrest if not rapidly terminated and hospital treatment is always indicated. Pending this, however, intravenous injection of lignocaine in a 100 mg bolus, or disopyramide 10 mg should be administered.

Ventricular dysrhythmic problems and syncope (margin)

Bradycardia

In a profound bradycardia, even though stroke volume may be good, cardiac output will be low and impair cerebral perfusion. Bradycardia is a feature of the common vaso-vagal or simple fainting state but may also be due to some drugs, particularly the ß-blockers, some illnesses, pain, and after myocardial infarction.

In the acute situation, intravenous atropine in a dose of

Bradycardia and syncope (margin)

0.6 mg is the treatment of choice. If bradycardia is persistent and chronic, drugs such as long acting isoprenaline (Saventrine) may be of benefit.

Sick sinus or 'tachy-brady' syndrome

Intermittent tachycardia and bradycardia

This difficult condition causes alternating tachycardia and bradycardia and is usually due to disease of the sinoatrial node. The only satisfactory treatment if the situation is severe is to suppress the tachycardia with ß-blockers and protect the patient from profound bradycardia by a permanent pacemaker.

Heart block

In this condition, the normal impulses from the atria are not conducted to the ventricles which therefore cannot respond.

Complete heart block causing Stokes – Adams attacks

There is a varying degree of block with a low or variable heart rate. If the block becomes complete, the ventricle assumes its own and usually very slow rhythm. This can result in long periods of little or no ventricular activity at all, and can cause syncope or partial syncope.

If there is any *impairment of consciousness* at all, *cardiac pacing is indicated.*

As an emergency measure, atropine 0.6 mg or isoprenaline may be tried intravenously.

Valvular heart disease

Diseased valves and low output

Any severe *valve lesion* which results in *low cardiac output* can cause impaired consciousness. The classical valve lesion to cause this is *aortic stenosis* and if a patient is having syncopal attacks or collapses, and has an aortic ejection systolic murmur, he should be referred for urgent consideration of aortic valve surgery.

Other valve lesions such as *tight mitral stenosis* or severe *aortic regurgitation* may lead to syncope due to a very low output state. A valve defect resulting in severe *pulmonary hypertension* may cause the same for the same reason. A rare but particularly important association between *mitral valve disease* and a *ball valve thrombus* may lead to abrupt loss of consciousness when the thrombus occludes the mitral valve. The same mechanism may occur in *left atrial myxoma.*

Congenital heart disease

Cyanotic heart disease

The diagnosis of syncope due to severe cyanotic heart disease is usually obvious and anoxic syncope may occur in situations with right to left shunting, particularly in Fallot's tetralogy. This is likely to occur in situations when the pulmonary infundibulum shuts down and so increases the right to left shunt.

Hypotension

Postural hypotension

Low blood pressure and syncope

Some normal persons have low blood pressures, and sudden changes of posture from sitting to lying positions to standing may be associated with a fall of systemic pressure with resultant faintness or syncope.

Postural hypotension caused by drugs

Any cause of low blood pressure may be associated with syncope but postural hypotension is commonly found with certain drugs such as the ganglion blockers or peripheral adrenergic inhibitors used in hypertension, the nitrites, histamine and levo-dopa.

Cerebral symptoms from changes of blood pressure are likely to occur when there is pre-existing cerebrovascular insufficiency such as vertebro-basilar or carotid disease and insufficiency.

Other low output states

Apart from valvular heart disease cardiac output may be poor due to a damaged myocardium.

Other causes of low cardiac output

It is not uncommon to find a history of transient syncope in patients who have sustained myocardial infarcts. This may be due to transient dysrhythmias but perfusion of tissue may be very poor after acute muscle damage. An increase in vaso-vagal state is found after inferior infarction and this reaction is potentiated by the use of opiates and relieved by intravenous atropine.

Effect of infarction

The cardiomyopathies will lead to low output states and may be associated with syncope.

Pulmonary embolism

Pulmonary embolism

While small pulmonary emboli are unlikely to be associated with impaired consciousness, a massive embolism occluding two-thirds of the pulmonary circulation is likely to cause collapse and syncope.

Cardiac compression

Constriction in compression of the heart

Decompensation of the heart will occur in situations when the heart is compressed either by severe constriction of the pericardium or by a large quantity of fluid in the pericardial space (cardiac tamponade). The former may occur in constrictive pericarditis (tuberculous, post-viral or collagen disease) and the latter in effusions due to infection, heart failure or malignant infiltration of the pericardium, or after infarction. The signs are gross with marked jugular venous elevation which increases on inspiration (Kussmaul's sign) or a pulse that is poor and diminishes or disappears on inspiration (pulsus paradoxus). This situation is an emergency that warrants urgent treatment.

Summary

Cardiac causes of syncope are common and include congenital and acquired heart disease, low output states and dysrhythmias and valvular disease as well as the many causes of hypotension.

Breathlessness

Presenting symptoms – Acute cardiac failure – Chronic heart failure – The signs of heart failure – Investigations in cardiac failure – Treatment of cardiac failure

Presenting symptoms

Breathlessness occurring at rest, with exertion or as deterioration of exercise tolerance. It may be mild and chronic or acute and severe.

Pulmonary and cardiac causes of breathlessness

A careful history from the patient will usually give a lead to the likelihood that the symptom of breathlessness is due to a cardiac cause. Organic pulmonary disease as a cause of breathlessness is suggested by symptoms, e.g. infected sputum, fever, pleuritic pain, a history of asthmatic bronchitis with wheezing, and examination of the chest together with chest X-ray will probably provide the answer.

The cardiac causes of breathlessness are likely to present as acute or chronic breathlessness, i.e. acute or chronic heart failure, pericardial effusions or constriction. It is fallacious to consider the two sides of the heart as failing independently for the heart usually will fail as an entire organ.

Nevertheless the concepts of right and left sided failure are well established because of the different clinical pictures that they produce.

61

Acute cardiac failure

Left ventricular failure

The features of acute heart failure

The history in acute left ventricular failure is characteristic. There is acute breathlessness which may come on at rest and is particularly likely to occur when the patient is in bed at night *(paroxysmal nocturnal dyspnoea)*. He wakes from sleep acutely distressed and breathless, feels the need to sit up or get up, and often goes to an open window for air.

Orthopnoea, breathlessness when lying flat, is another important symptom and is often noticed after the patient starts the night propped up on pillows which he later slides off and comes to lie flat. This will lead to increased venous return to the lungs which will lead to pulmonary congestion in lungs that are already overloaded from an increased pulmonary venous pressure from poor left ventricular function.

Haemo-dynamics of left ventricular failure

In left ventricular failure, the ventricle fails to discharge its contents adequately with a resultant rise in end diastolic pressure and pulmonary venous pressure. This in turn causes venous pooling in the lungs and fluid from the blood, a transudate, may pass from pulmonary capillaries into the alveolar air cells. This fluid will impede gaseous exchange and cause acute breathlessness (pulmonary oedema).

The increased pulmonary venous pressure may be transmitted backwards to pulmonary arteries and the right side of the heart which may in turn become strained. The signs of right sided failure may ensue and when right sided failure follows on left, it is known as congestive cardiac failure.

Congestive cardiac failure

There may be some compensation for left ventricular failure by this process of pooling blood in the lungs, transudation, and venous pooling in the liver.

Acute right ventricular failure

Acute right sided heart failure

As an entity on its own, right ventricular failure is much rarer than the features of right ventricular failure that are found in congestive failure (ie total heart failure or right following on left ventricular failure).

The symptoms of right ventricular failure are less pronounced because the lungs are not overloaded. Dyspnoea will occur because the pulmonary arterial input to the lungs is not adequate to maintain sufficient arterial oxygen saturation.

Apart from a milder degree of breathlessness the patient will notice *undue fatiguability, lethargy and heaviness of the limbs* due to venous pooling. Congestion of the liver or stomach may lead to *nausea and vomiting.*

Causes of acute cardiac failure

	Left	Right
The main causes of left and right sided failure	Hypertension	Pulmonary hypertension and cor pulmonale
	Aortic valve disease	
	Mitral regurgitation	Pulmonary embolism
	Cardiomyopathies	Pulmonary valve disease
	Myocardial infarction	Tricuspid valve disease
	Coronary artery disease	
	Acute dysrhythmia	

The causes that have been listed are the commoner ones that are associated with *low output heart failure,* which by definition is that state when *ventricular output is inadequate to oxygenate the organs that it provides.*

High output failure   There are causes of *high output* state cardiac failure such as:

Thyrotoxicosis

Anaemia

Beri-beri

Hypoxic cor pulmonale

Features of high output failure   When cardiac output is high, the heart may fail because of excessive demands put on it. The signs of cardiac failure will be present with evidence of raised output, dilated and throbbing digital vessels and a warm periphery.

Haemo-dynamic changes in heart failure   The causes of heart failure that have been listed all result in diminished myocardial function by one means or another. Hypertension, aortic valve disease and mitral regurgitation cause increased cardiac work to maintain the cardiac output. This causes left ventricular hypertrophy or in the case of aortic regurgitation, dilatation. After a phase of compensation, the left ventricular muscle bulk outgrows its vascular supply and the muscle begins to fail. When this happens the left ventricular diastolic pressure rises and this pressure rise is transmitted back via the left atrium, to the lungs. As has been mentioned, acute episodes of fluid transudation into the lungs will cause acute pulmonary oedema, an emergency situation when the patient is acutely breathless and distressed feeling that he is suffocating or drowning, which indeed he is, and may cough copious amounts of frothy, pink sputum or develop a marked wheeze (*cardiac asthma*).

Cardio-
myopathies
and heart
failure

The cardiomyopathies are caused by various types of organic disease, e.g. amyloidosis, alcohol, haemochromatosis, diabetes mellitus and collagen disorders. The most usual manifestation of the *cardiomyopathies* is as *congestive cardiac failure*. In this situation it is primary disease of the muscle itself which causes it to fail. In the same way *coronary artery disease* may cause heart failure by causing brown atrophy of cardiac muscle when angina may not be a frequent manifestation, the patient presenting with heart failure.

When myocardial infarction is the cause of heart failure it is usually acute and will be obvious from the history. This is certainly so in younger groups but great suspicion about the possibility of infarction must be raised when an *elderly person* presents with *acute breathlessness* due to heart failure. The older age groups not infrequently sustain infarcts which are painless, the so-called '*silent infarcts*', but present as acute left ventricular failure.

Pure right sided heart failure is caused by lesions affecting the right side of the heart primarily and so causes right ventricular hypertrophy and strain and thence failure. Congestive heart failure as has already been mentioned is the succession of right heart failure following on from left.

Chronic heart failure

Heart failure
becoming
chronic

In any of the causes of heart failure that have been considered, a chronic state of failure may be reached. Chronicity will be due to the lesions and causes that have been named, producing a more persistent and less severe picture. That is, breathlessness is probably slight becoming moderate or severe with exertion, and the signs of heart failure are mild but persistent.

Symptoms of
chronic
failure

Apart from breathlessness attributable to chronically stiff lungs due to congestion, the patient will complain of fatiguability because of diminished cardiac output, and heaviness and tiredness of the limbs due to swollen and congested limbs. In addition chronic congestion of the stomach may cause anorexia and nausea, and swelling of the liver stretches the capsule and may cause discomfort. Inadequate or partial treatment of acute failure or treatment of a severe state of failure may lead to modification and a chronic state of failure.

The signs of heart failure

Physical signs
of acute left
ventricular
failure

The cardinal signs of heart failure must be looked for in any patient presenting with breathlessness. In *acute left ventricular failure* the patient will appear breathless and anxious. The breathlessness may be due to pulmonary oedema when the patient is extremely distressed producing frothy pink sputum, cardiac asthma when there is wheezing due to narrowing of the bronchi from bronchial oedema, orthopnoea, or Cheyne-Stokes respiration.

The pulse pressure is small and may be of alternans type, and increased adrenergic activity causes peripheral pallor, cold extremeties and sweating. The blood pressure initially may be elevated due to peripheral vasoconstriction and constriction of the renal arteries.

Heart sounds

On *auscultation* of the heart a triple rhythm due to either a third or fourth heart sound is heard which if associated with a tachycardia produces a *gallop rhythm.* The third heart sound is associated with left ventricular rapid filling which may occur in most causes of heart failure. This sound occurs shortly after aortic valve closure and is best heard at the apex or with the patient lying in the left lateral position.

A fourth heart sound may be heard when either ventricle is stressed, and increased atrial contraction is necessary to increase left ventricular end diastolic pressure. This causes the fourth heart sound which when associated with a tachycardia, produces a pre-systolic gallop rhythm. Auscultation of the lung fields is likely to reveal fine rales or crepitations on both sides; if due to pulmonary oedema, the crepitations are likely to be widespread.

In *right ventricular failure* the cardinal signs are usually obvious and are:

Cardinal signs
of right heart
failure

(i) Elevation of the jugular venous pressure,
(ii) Hepatomegaly,
(iii) Oedema (lower limbs and sacral).

The same signs will be evident in *congestive cardiac failure* when the signs of left ventricular failure will be present as well.

The jugular venous pressure is measured by examining the neck with the patient laying semi-recumbent at 45 degrees. The liver is palpated in the normal way and pressure applied on the liver may result in increase of jugular venous pressure, the hepato-jugular reflux.

Problems in cardiology

In congestive failure it may be possible to demonstrate ascites, pleural effusions or a pericardial effusion. When the signs of failure are seen, the possibility of a pericardial effusion must be borne in mind which will cause breathlessness and mimic failure.

Investigations in cardiac failure

Value of chest X-ray in heart failure

The key investigations in the diagnosis of heart failure are a chest X-ray and electrocardiograph.

The chest X-ray is taken to show the following features:

(i) Cardiomegaly and an increased cardio-thoracic ratio,
(ii) The contours of the cardiac silhouette,
(iii) The presence of pulmonary venous congestion,
(iv) Fluid in the fissures,
(v) Pleural effusions.

Most of these features will be found in congestive cardiac failure and will give strong clues that the cause of breathlessness is cardiac in origin. The most reliable signs on the chest X-ray of early heart failure will be enlargement of the heart and congestion of the upper lobe veins. The very earliest sign of congestion is when the upper lobe veins are seen to be equal in diameter to the lower lobe veins. Usually, because of the effect of gravity, their diameter is smaller.

As failure becomes more florid the changes on X-ray become more marked until gross venous congestion produces the classical batswing appearance with interstitial oedema and effusions.

Electrocardiograph

Electro-cardiograph changes and heart failure

This is not pathognomonic of heart failure in any way but is likely to give a clue that heart disease is present.

In some cases of unexplained failure, when the e.c.g. may show the presence of a contributory dysrhythmia, it is not by any means uncommon to find the onset of rapid atrial fibrillation as a cause of heart failure.

It is important, particularly in the elderly, to exclude myocardial infarction as a cause of sudden failure. The e.c.g. may also show the presence of coronary artery disease, an ischaemic pattern, although the anginal symptoms of coronary disease may be absent.

Breathlessness

The e.c.g. may show left ventricular hypertrophy and strain which may be due to hypertension, aortic valve disease or mitral regurgitation. It may also show unusual patterns such as abnormalities of the QRS complexes in various types of cardiomyopathy.

It is helpful therefore, not in being diagnostic of heart failure, but in showing that some form of cardiac disease is present.

Other investigations

Important investigations and heart failure

Apart from actually making a diagnosis of heart failure a cause must always be sought and found. This is important because of the possibility of detecting correctable causes such as valvular disease, thyrotoxicosis or anaemia. A clue as to the actual cause of failure is very likely to have arisen from careful history taking and examination. It must be remembered that even mild anaemia may tip the balance in a person who has a predisposition to failure for other reasons.

Thyrotoxicosis may not be very evident, particularly in the elderly, and must be suspected if atrial fibrillation is present and is unexplained. Other investigations that should be undertaken are the blood sugar to exclude diabetes, and blood cultures to exclude endocarditis in a patient who has a valvular defect, and worsening and unexplained failure associated with a fever.

Treatment of cardiac failure

As has already been described, there are various clinical pictures of cardiac failure that may be encountered and the management and treatment of them will be described.

Acute left ventricular failure

In its severest form acute left ventricular failure may be manifest as pulmonary oedema. This should be treated as a medical emergency but vital measures must be taken pending hospital admission. The following general care measures should be adhered to.

General care

(i) The patient should rest and be propped sitting up.

(ii) Oxygen should be administered if possible.

Problems in cardiology

Drugs

The following drugs should be given.

(i) Intravenous frusemide 40 mg (or i.m.) or bumetanide 1 mg iv.

(ii) Intravenous aminophylline 0.25–0.5 g, given slowly to avoid dysrhythmias.

(iii) Digitalization. The first dose of digoxin 0.5 mg may be given intravenously if the patient is not receiving digoxin. Alternatively the loading dose may be given by intramuscular injection. Digoxin is effective in sinus rhythm or atrial fibrillation, tachycardia or bradycardia.

(iv) Morphine or diamorphine. Morphine may be given in a dose of 15 mg intramuscularly or 10 mg intravenously. Alternatively diamorphine 2.5–10 mg i.v. or i.m. may be given. These drugs are very beneficial in that they prevent hyperventilation and relieve the extreme anxiety that is so manifest. Caution should be observed in patients who have chronic obstructive airways disease lest repiratory depression is extreme with resultant apnoea (if this occurs it should be countered quickly with intravenous nalorphine).

Physical measures in managing left ventricular failure

Benefit may be obtained by cuffing the limbs alternately, particularly by cuffing thighs and inflating the sphygmomanometer to just above the venous pressure. This will cause venous pooling in the limbs and so diminish pulmonary venous congestion.

The removal of 500 ml of blood from the venous system may be very effective and result in dramatic improvement.

If there are facilities to suck out the airway, removal of frothy oedema fluid from the airways is beneficial and may be undertaken in hospital under bronchoscopy.

Positive pressure ventilation is very effective in hospital in producing better oxygenation and by forcing oedema fluid back from the alveolar air cells into the circulation.

Treatment in less acute failure

Once the patient with acute left ventricular or congestive cardiac failure is beginning to stabilize, maintenance therapy should be instituted.

Key drugs in the treatment of acute left ventricular failure (margin)

Cuffing (margin)

Venesection (margin)

Suction (margin)

Ventilation (margin)

Management when failure is stabilized (margin)

68

Breathlessness

The patient should be nursed in bed, preferably a cardiac bed or chair, so that the legs are dependent, and oxygen should be administered.

Drugs

Digitalis
In spite of the fact that modern diuretics such as frusemide and bumetanide are extremely potent and will alone often relieve pulmonary oedema, patients should be fully digitalized. After the loading dose of 0.5 mg digoxin either i.m. or i.v. the maintenance dose must be judged carefully according to age and size. The *elderly are often very sensitive to digitalis* which should be given with caution. In general, digoxin in a dose of 0.25 mg is given either orally or intramuscularly eight hourly until the heart rate falls or nausea develops. In the presence of hypokalaemia, patients, particularly the elderly, are much more sensitive to digitalis. Contrarily, some will need 0.5 mg digoxin eight hourly for one to two days before full digitalization is achieved. If the patient is in atrial fibrillation, the response must be monitored by measuring the rate at the apex.

Serum digoxin levels
If the facility is available, the serum digoxin level can be measured to check that the dosage has achieved the therapeutic range 0.8–1.8 ng/l. The benefits of digitalis cannot be overstressed and usual maintenance dosage is 0.25 mg b.d. though the elderly may need much smaller doses than this, using multiples of the paediatric tablet, 0.0625 mg.

Use of digitalis in spite of potent diuretics
In spite of the potency of modern diuretic therapy, and although in the treatment of acute heart failure drugs such as frusemide will often suffice in relieving the symptoms and severe distress, digitalis has an important place. This is particularly so in maintenance therapy, in diminishing the need for diuretic therapy to maintain equilibrium and in allowing the use of a less potent and hence perhaps a potassium-sparing diuretic, an important factor in the elderly.

Toxic effects of digitalis
But care must be exercised in using digitalis drugs for they have toxicity, and apart from nausea and vomiting they may be cardio-toxic, inducing some supraventricular dysrhythmias. Ventricular extrasystoles may herald more important and dangerous ventricular tachycardias.

Ideally the therapeutic level of digitalis dosage should be confirmed by serum levels, but failing this, a dose should be used below that which will produce nausea, and the appearance of ventricular extrasystoles or other dysrhythmias will certainly indicate temporary cessation of the drug.

69

α-blocking drugs

With the advent of other types of treatment for heart failure, notably the α-blocking drugs hydralazine and Rogitine which are currently in vogue in some types of hospital practice when digitalis drugs are out of fashion, the *benefits of digitalis remain extremely important* particularly to patients being treated in general practice and on an out-patient basis.

Diuretic maintenance therapy

Having treated the acute stage of heart failure, the general principle of treatment should be to reduce the dose of diuretics to the lowest level that allows compensation of cardiac failure and in achieving this, to use the least potent diuretic that will do so. In short this means that whereas the most potent diuretics such as frusemide (Lasix) or bumetanide (Burinex) are necessary in the treatment of acute heart failure, once stabilization and compensation have reached, a less potent diuretic such as a thiazide or any other longer and smoother acting diuretic should be substituted. This does not alter the fact that some patients with more severe and persistent heart failure, where no remedial course is possible, may need high potency diuretic treatment to maintain a state of compensated failure. In, for example, severe inoperable valvular disease of the heart, or an untreatable congestive cardiomyopathy, it is not unusual to use a twice daily regime of a drug such as frusemide. But an attempt must always be made to reduce the amount of diuretic treatment to a maintenance level in order that there is a reserve of armamentarium, or 'shots in the locker' available if the situation deteriorates again.

Increasing diuretic therapy

Having discussed the changes advocated when improvement takes place it is equally important to be prepared to 'tighten' diuretic treatment if it does not. If cardiac failure is persistent and appears to become intractable, maximum doses of the most potent diuretics must be used and advantage taken of the synergism that exists between the ordinary thiazide type diuretics and those such as spironolactone, triamterene and amiloride. First of all it is always worthwhile to quickly ring the changes lest the patient has become resistant to one particular diuretic, e.g. frusemide. If a patient no longer appears to respond to, for example, frusemide, it is well worth changing first to bumetanide (Burinex) or ethacrynic acid or metalozol (Metenix). Failing this, spironolactone (an aldosterone antagonist) should be added to the regime starting in a dose of 25 mg t.d.s. The benefit will not be immediate and may take several days to provoke a diuresis. The addition of this drug will lessen or remove the need for concurrent

Resistance to diuretics

Secondary
hyper-
aldosteronism

potassium therapy as it is a potassium conserver, like both triamterene and amiloride. Some patients with chronic congestive failure, particularly when tricuspid valve disease is present, develop secondary hyperaldosteronism and respond well to spironolactone. If possible this drug should not be used in the long term unless the situation is intractable (as in secondary aldosteronism) when it may be necessary. Spironolactone (Aldactone) not uncommonly produces the side effects of nausea and the male particularly may notice gynaecomastia and soreness of breast tissue.

When intractable heart failure does not respond to the above measures, treatment in hospital is indicated. It must be remembered that bed rest, salt restriction and careful observation of compliance to treatment are very important factors, and that in hospital other therapy is now possible which needs haemodynamic monitoring not available in domiciliary practice. In addition such important measures as electrolyte control, so necessary and vital with large doses of different diuretics, must be exercised. When severe electrolyte disorder exists, for example a marked hyponatraemia, a patient may become resistant to all diuretics.

Long-term management

Assuming that correctable causes of heart failure have been sought and when appropriate have been corrected, the problem often remains of long-term maintenance. Trial will prove that in many cases it is possible to wean patients off diuretics and digitalis preparations over a period of weeks or months. In many patients, long-term benefit may accrue from the use of digitalis in a dose appropriate to age and size, for its positive inotropism leads to increased cardiac output which in turn has a diuretic effect.

General advice as to weight reduction where appropriate, restriction of salt intake and exercise and a life style that are appropriate to the patient's condition can really be only assessed in individual cases.

With modern therapy, the prognosis of heart failure, even in a patient who has presented in acute left ventricular failure for an unremedial cause, is a very different one from ten or twenty years ago and now many live reasonable lives for some years in a state of cardiac compensation.

Conclusion

A remedial cause must be sought before accepting that conventional anti-failure treatment must be maintained. For example, has the post-infarction patient in persistent failure developed a left ventricular aneurysm or a ventricular septal defect due to infarcted septum? Is there any evidence of valvular disease or endocarditis superimposed on pre-existing valvular disease? Is there myocardial infarction (often painless in the elderly)?

These questions are of the utmost importance and answers may only be forthcoming from shrewd assessment and history taking, and relatively simple investigations, before any specialized methods of investigation are warranted.

In spite of the advent of potent and effective diuretics digitalis has an important place in treatment. Particular care must be exercised in using digitalis with diuretics which cause potassium loss. Hypokalaemia may enhance digitalis toxicity.

7 Infective and invasive processes of the heart

Pericardium – Myocardium – Endocardium

Presentation

Fever of unexplained cause. Chest pain of pericarditic type or pleuro-pericarditis. Unexplained heart failure. Cardiac tamponade or pericardial constriction masquerading as heart failure.

Involvement of the heart by metastases, collagen disorders, or infective organisms, may occur in any of the three main layers of the heart.

(i) Pericardium,
(ii) Myocardium,
(iii) Endocardium.

Involvement of the pericardium by any process may present as pericarditic pain, or breathlessness due to effusion or constriction.

Pericardium
Pericarditis

Pain of pericarditis

This condition is not uncommon and is most usually due to infection with a virus usually the Coxsackie type B virus. It may present as chest pain hence its important differentiation from the pain of myocardial ischaemia or infarction. Pericarditis may also occur in certain bacterial infections as a complication of pneumonia and pleurisy, lung abscesses or mediastinitis.

73

Tuberculous pericarditis is rarer, but pericardial involvement is seen as a complication of collagen disorders, notably disseminated lupus erythematosus or Still's disease in children or adolescents. It may also occur as a complication of rheumatic fever.

Pericarditic pain

Pain of
pericarditis

The pain of pericarditis is usually very sharp and severe. It is central and may radiate to the jaw or shoulder but its most diagnostic feature is that it is positional and postural, that is relief or exacerbation are noticed by sitting forward, lying back or turning on one side or another. The pain may also be influenced by respiration and change in intensity during different phases of respiration.

Pericardial effusions

Effusions and
pericarditis

Tamponade

Effusions may develop in any form of pericardial involvement and where the two surfaces of the pericardium are separated by fluid, pain is a less likely feature. The patient will present with breathlessness, elevated jugular venous pressure and congestion which may lead on to the most severe form, tamponade, an emergency situation when the pulse is of very poor volume exhibiting a paradoxical nature, that is, diminishing in volume on inspiration with the jugular venous pressure being seen to rise on inspiration (Kussmaul's sign). In addition there may be ascites and hepatic enlargement. Pericarditis presenting as a large effusion is more likely to be due to malignant metastatic spread, tuberculosis or uraemia, than due to the viral or so called non-specific types of pericarditis.

Differentiation
between a
large heart,
cardiomegaly
or effusion

In practice, the problem that exists and is of the utmost importance is to differentiate marked cardiomegaly due to or as a cause of heart failure from a large heart shadow due to an effusion. This may need specialized type of investigation by catheterization, fluoroscopy, echocardiography, or isotope scanning, and because of the very different therapeutic implications, investigation is of a great importance.

Therefore the question must always be asked with respect to any patient who has presented in failure, and in whom chest X-ray has revealed a large heart silhouette, *'could this be an effusion that warrants further urgent investigation?'*

Pericardial constriction

Constrictive pericarditis is much less common as tuberculosis has become less common. Tuberculous infection of the pericardium usually from mediastinal lymph node spread, may lead to constriction of the pericardium. Other less common causes of constriction are viral pericarditis and collagen disease. The features that lead to suspicion of constrictive pericarditis are:

(i) Breathlessness,

(ii) Elevated jugular venous pressure which rises on inspiration,

(iii) A small pulse volume that diminishes on inspiration, ascites, oedema of the lower limbs and a *small* heart shadow in contrast to an effusion, an X-ray of which penetrated with oblique or lateral views may show the presence of calcification if of tuberculous aetiology.

Viral pericarditis

This condition is seen commonly, often in small epidemics, in young adults and the middle-aged.

Features of viral pericarditis
Before the pain presents there is usually the characteristic prodromal illness of a viral infection with fever, malaise, sore throat and perhaps cough. This is not always so and some cases present with the typical pain that has already been described.

Usually at some point of the illness, a pericardial rub will be heard but this may be transitory. The ESR is usually elevated and the most helpful investigation is the e.c.g. which shows concave ST elevation, which due to the nature of the generalized pericarditic inflammation is not confined to any particular vascular distribution pattern as is seen in ischaemic heart disease.

Salicylates
The disease runs a course of several days or a few weeks but has a tendency for relapse to occur. There is good response to bed rest, and salicylates should be given in full dosage four time per day. If relapses do occur or the condition is slow to
Steroids
respond to salicylates, corticosteroids are extremely effective as they are in the pericarditis of post-infarction or Dressler's syndrome. Prednisolone is given at a starting dose of 45 mg per day reducing and tailing off the drug as clinical improvement is seen. Once a patient has had an attack of pericarditis, there is an increased tendency for recurrence in later years.

The immediate complications of pericarditis are occasional dysrhythmias and pericardial effusions. A possible but late sequel to the infection is the development of constriction.

Other types of pericarditis

Collagen disease

Pericarditic pain is a feature of conditions such as disseminated lupus erythematosus often in association with pleuritic pain and pleural and pericardial effusions. The diagnosis will be supported by a high ESR, the detection of LE cells in the blood together with the other clinical features of disseminated lupus erythematosus.

Uraemic pericarditis

In chronic renal failure, uraemic pericarditis may develop as the blood urea rises to levels usually above 30 mmol/l. A pericardial rub may be heard and the patient becomes breathless as an effusion develops with probable associated anaemia.

Tuberculous pericarditis

Acid-fast bacillus infection must be considered in any case of pericarditis that presents when the aetiology is not clear. The diagnosis may be suggested by the clinical picture, Mantoux test and examination of pericardial fluid.

In cases where doubt exists, a trial of conventional antituberculous drugs may be justified.

Malignancy

Pericarditis is often found in spread from carcinoma of the bronchus or breast. While pain may be a feature, effusion and possible tamponade are more common.

Myocardium

A variety of pathological processes may affect the myocardium and result in a group of conditions known as the cardiomyopathies.

In practice, the most usual way that the cardiomyopathies present is as congestive cardiac failure and such conditions as sarcoidosis, haemochromatosis, amyloidosis, malnutrition, alcoholism and the post-partum state are examples of processes that result in myocardial cell damage and heart failure.

The heart muscle cells may also degenerate in myxoedema

and thyrotoxicosis, acromegaly, certain types of muscular dystrophy and Friedreich's ataxia and other congenital causes. This group of conditions has to be considered in any case of heart failure when the cause is not obvious.

Myocarditis

Myocardial inflammation

Inflammatory conditions of the myocardium are usually less difficult to diagnose as they present as part of an illness which may be viral, bacterial, collagen disease, rheumatic, allergic, toxic, parasitic or fungal in origin.

Viral myocarditis is not uncommonly seen as a complication of pericarditis. This is likely to be due to the Coxsackie B virus but also can occur as a complication of glandular fever, mumps and poliomyelitis. It may also be found in infective hepatitis and viral pneumonia. If looked for, myocarditis is perhaps not altogether uncommon as a complication of such simple infections as the common cold and influenza.

In viral infections, the patient with myocarditis as a complication of a generalized infection may show the signs of heart failure but the diagnosis may only be established by auscultation of the heart when a triple or gallop rhythm is heard and by showing characteristic e.c.g. changes.

Usually viral myocarditis will resolve spontaneously but anti-failure treatment may need to be instituted and consideration given to the use of steroids. Some cases of Coxsackie myocarditis have been fatal.

Viral peri- and myocarditis are much commoner than is thought and will be diagnosed if looked for in the patient presenting with a febrile 'flu-like' illness, particularly if there is any evidence of heart failure or an unexplained gallop rhythm.

Rheumatic myocarditis

Rheumatic myocarditis

This condition is extremely important to diagnose in a patient with rheumatic fever. The fact that the heart is involved in rheumatic fever will influence treatment at the time and will accentuate the importance of follow up. It is diagnosed by the appearance of cardiac murmurs during the course of rheumatic fever, abnormal e.c.gs with dysrhythmias and conduction defects, and a tachycardia out of keeping with the degree of fever.

Collagen disorder

Collagen
disease

The myocardium may become involved in collagen disease such as systemic lupus of polyarteritis nodosa and will be suspected when heart failure is evident, with abnormal e.c.gs and a gallop rhythm present.

Toxic myocarditis

Any severe toxic state such as overwhelming infection or septicaemia can cause myocarditis leading to heart failure. This will often resolve with treatment of the underlying condition.

Endocardium
Endocarditis

It is important to be aware of the possibility of infective endocarditis in any patient with known rheumatic or congenital heart disease who presents with the *vague symptoms of malaise, fever, lethargy and tiredness, and weight loss.* In fact the symptoms are often like those of febrile influenza-like illnesses and are non-specific in their presentation. *Aortic regurgitation* and *mitral regurgitation* are the most susceptible valve lesions.

Bacterial endocarditis

Bacterial
involvement of
the endo-
cardium

This is the commonest form of endocarditis and presents in a sub-acute and acute form. In the elderly a chronic form has been described. In *sub-acute bacterial endocarditis* the most usual infecting organism is a *β*-haemolytic streptococcus *(Streptococcus viridans)*. Infection with this organism may follow dental treatment of any form, extractions, fillings or scaling, when penicillin or other antibiotic cover has not been given. Other organisms are also found as causes, e.g. *E. coli, Streptococcus faecalis*, and may complicate infections in *any other parts of the body, surgery or instrumentation of the genito-urinary or gastrointestinal tract without antiobiotic cover.*

Presentation of endocarditis

Suspicion of endocarditis should be aroused in any patient with a cardiac murmur, particularly of an incompetent valve, who presents with an *unexplained febrile illness*, anaemia, lethargy, weight loss, joint pains or deterioration of cardiac function.

The following physical signs should be looked for.

Splinter haemorrhages

These may be seen in the nails and are particularly significant in the proximal two-thirds of the nail (the outer part of the nail often shows these due to trauma of work). They may also be seen in the fundi, the conjunctivae, skin or mucous membrane. Under the nail, they look like small spinters and are particularly significant when of reddish hue.

Clubbing of fingers

This takes at least six weeks to develop and will be seen in about half of all cases of sub-acute endocarditis. Clubbing is also seen in the toes.

Nodes

Tender pink painful lumps are found in the finger or toe pads. They fade to a bluish colour and are due to cutaneous emboli (Osler's nodes).

Splenomegaly

This is common and is not usually massive unless splenic infarction takes place.

Skin changes

'Cafe au lait' spots are seen very rarely. Petechial haemorrhages are much more common, and are due to capillary haemorrhage, or a capillaritis. Osler's nodes are painful small lumps in the finger pulps.

Emboli

These may occur anywhere but may present as pulmonary embolism when infective vegetations embolise from the site of a septal defect with left to right heart shunting e.g. ventricular septal defect.

79

Complications of sub-acute bacterial endocarditis

Deterioration of cardiac function

Complications   A valve lesion may deteriorate rapidly once a bacterial infection is established and may cause heart failure. This is particularly so in regurgitant lesions when the murmur is noticed to change.

Mycotic aneurysms

Bacteria infect and destroy arterial wall tissue and cause an aneurysm which may rupture and bleed and prove fatal if in the cerebral circulation, when it may present as a catastrophic stroke.

Renal complications

    (a) Renal infarction or haematuria
    (b) Embolic focal nephritis
    (c) Diffuse glomerulonephritis – renal failure
    (d) Abscess formation due to bacteraemia
    (e) Renal congestion – albuminuria and red cells.

Ocular complications

    (a) Loss or partial loss or vision due to embolism
    (b) Petechiae of retina
    (c) Papilloedema or papillitis is found with diffuse glomerulonephritis.

Investigations for sub-acute bacterial endocarditis

Important investigations in SBE

    (i) Full blood picture and sedimentation rate. There will often be a mild degree of anaemia, slight leucocytosis and elevation of the ESR.

    (ii) Examination of urine. Urine should be examined microscopically on at least three occasions for the presence of red blood cells due to micro-emboli.

    (iii) The keystone of investigation is blood culture. This should if necessary be undertaken on at least four different occasions and will be most likely to give a positive culture when fever is present.

These investigations may be started by the family physician in screening a patient for endocarditis, or prior to hospital referral.

Treatment of sub-acute bacterial endocarditis

This will usually be undertaken in hospital or certainly in conjunction with a hospital physician. The antibiotic(s) used will depend on the infecting organism.

Antibiotics

Streptococcus viridans will usually respond and be sensitive to penicillin and will require a minimum of four and up to twelve mega-units per day, preferably given intravenously.

With other organisms one will rely on the use of ampicillin, cloxacillin or the cephalosporins. When an organism has not been isolated by culture and the decision has been made to treat on clinical grounds, penicillin in a dose of up to 30 mega-units per day with the addition of gentamicin is a useful regime of fairly wide spectrum.

The duration of treatment is usually in the region of six weeks and although clinical response will usually be seen much earlier, treatment should continue for longer to lessen the chance of relapse.

Preventive treatment

Prophylaxis

(i) All patients with *rheumatic* and *congenital heart disease* undergoing *dental treatment* in the form of *extractions*, *fillings* or *scaling*, must have *penicillin* cover immediately before treatment and continuing for three days.

(ii) A patient with proven endocarditis must be examined by a dental surgeon and have the jaws and teeth X-rayed looking for caries and infected roots. If these are found and the patient is under treatment with antibiotics, a change of antibiotic during treatment is advisable.

It is always safer to err on the side of caution and treat a patient for endocarditis when there is reasonable clinical suspicion unsubstantiated by bacteriological tests lest the condition progresses with resultant ravaging of the infected valve.

Acute endocarditis

Acute infection

This condition is much more florid and easier to diagnose. The patient will be considerably more ill than in sub-acute endocarditis with fever, anaemia, skin rashes and often painful swollen joints.

Blood culture is almost invariably positive and the likely organism *Staphylococcus aureus*, or other pyogenic bacteria. Urgent treatment with the appropriate antibiotic is essential to prevent rapid deterioration of valve function and the condition carries a high morbidity and significant mortality.

Chronic endocarditis

Chronic infection

This is rare but has been more commonly described in the elderly and may run a long and fairly benign course. The features are mild and the diagnosis often difficult but must be considered in a patient with a cardiac lesion who has an unexplained fever. Blood cultures are often negative but it may be justified to try empirical treatment with antibiotics and observe the response. Occasionally bone marrow culture will be productive of an organism when conventional blood culture has failed.

Summary

Many common types of infection particularly viral, may cause peri- or myocarditis. If sought, these conditions are not rare.

The diagnosis of bacterial endocarditis is of paramount importance for if missed, it may result in catastrophic valve deterioration. It is safer to err on the side of caution and treat if the diagnosis is uncertain.

Electrocardiography

Particular value of the e.c.g. in practice – Reading and record-ing the e.c.g. – Some samples of common e.c.g. abnormalities

This does present a problem in practice because electrocardio-graphy is often misunderstood, misundertaken and misin-terpreted. It is essential that the family physician should either be proficient in understanding and interpreting the e.c.g. tracing he has obtained from his own apparatus, or should know the clear indications for referring a patient for an e.c.g. study at a hospital, and being able to include the information from it correctly in the clinical situation.

The problems of e.c.g.s in practice
Many family physicians now practising have had adequate training as junior hospital doctors or as interns, as to make them reasonably proficient to record an e.c.g. tracing and read it. Alternatively some have learned the harder way, by owning the equipment, using it frequently and from the help of books, articles, lectures and courses become proficient by practice. This is much more difficult, for to learn this way the doctor has to report and be responsible for reporting on a fairly large volume of tracings, which is not always easy in a busy practice, but is easier in hospital practice where he may be responsible for the reporting service on all e.c.g.s of that hospital.

If one has doubts about proficiency in interpreting an e.c.g., then this is a potentially dangerous situation and expert help should always be sought or perhaps better, the patient be referred to a specialist unit.

If however, the family physician is confident as to his skill in reading, interpreting and drawing the correct conclusion,

83

the equipment is of enormous value to the practice of good medicine, will give greater work satisfaction, and be an adjunct to diagnostic skills.

Particular value of the e.c.g. in practice

The e.c.g. may be of value:

Value of
the e.c.g.

(i) To record and diagnose a dysrhythmia when the patient complains of 'palpitations', bumping of the heart, missed beats or slow or rapid pulse.

(ii) To assess the state of left ventricular tissue, i.e. the presence of left ventricular hypertrophy and strain in such conditions as systemic hypertension, aortic and mitral valvular disease.

(iii) To assess the state of the myocardium in patients who have ischaemic heart disease presenting as angina. It must be remembered that the resting e.c.g. is often normal and the diagnosis of angina is essentially a clinical one, but the presence of ischaemic changes will aid the diagnosis.

Abnormal changes may be brought out by exercise or stress (exercise e.c.g.) which should only be undertaken when the facility for defibrillation is present.

(iv) In the diagnosis of myocardial infarction. Again, essentially a clinical diagnosis assessed by the type and duration of pain, the e.c.g. may prove a useful aid. The hazards of the e.c.g. in the diagnosis are:

Hazards of
e.c.g. diagnosis
of infarction

(a) That the e.c.g. may show no change in the early stages of infarction and may take 48 hours to show changes.

(b) That the changes are present but are overlooked by a non-proficient person.

(c) That the changes are long-standing and not new, and are not related to the current situation.

If infarction is suspected, either an e.c.g. should be recorded at the home or consulting room, or the patient admitted directly to a coronary unit. The patient must never be referred for an out-patient e.c.g. which will not be read and interpreted immediately by a doctor before the patient leaves hospital.

(d) In chest pain thought not to be of cardiac origin, e.g. neurosis or 'chest wall' pain. A patient who has non-cardiac pain but who is anxious may gain considerable reassurance from a normal e.c.g. record.

Reading and recording the e.c.g.

It is not appropriate in this text to give an account of the electrophysiology of the heart and a detailed account of how the activity of the conducting system of heart tissue is translated into an e.c.g. record. For this, reference should be made to a simple text book on electrocardiography.

Suffice it to say that cardiac muscle contraction is mediated by electrical activity spreading through a special conducting system by an excitatory process associated with depolarization and then repolarization. This changing process is recorded graphically as upward or downward deflections on the e.c.g. tracing.

The basic wave components of the e.c.g.

Spread of electrical impulse through the heart
The electrical impulse is initiated in the conducting system at the sino-atrial (S-A) node. It then spreads through atrial tissue to the atrio-ventricular (A-V) node. The impulse then passes down the special conducting systems via the bundle of His to the branches supplying right and left ventricles (the right and left bundles, the latter having two fascicles, anterior and posterior). It then spreads via the Purkinje fibres outward to the surface of the ventricles.

The main wave components of the e.c.g. tracing are the P, Q, R, S, and T waves.

P wave – represents atrial depolarization
Q wave – an initial negative downward
      deflection   ) Represent
R wave – the first upward deflection   ) ventricular
S wave – the first downward deflection) depolarization
      after R
T wave – ventricular repolarization.
      (Figure 8.1a)
U wave – not usually of significance

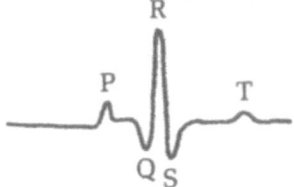

Figure 8.1a   The normal wave components of the e.c.g.

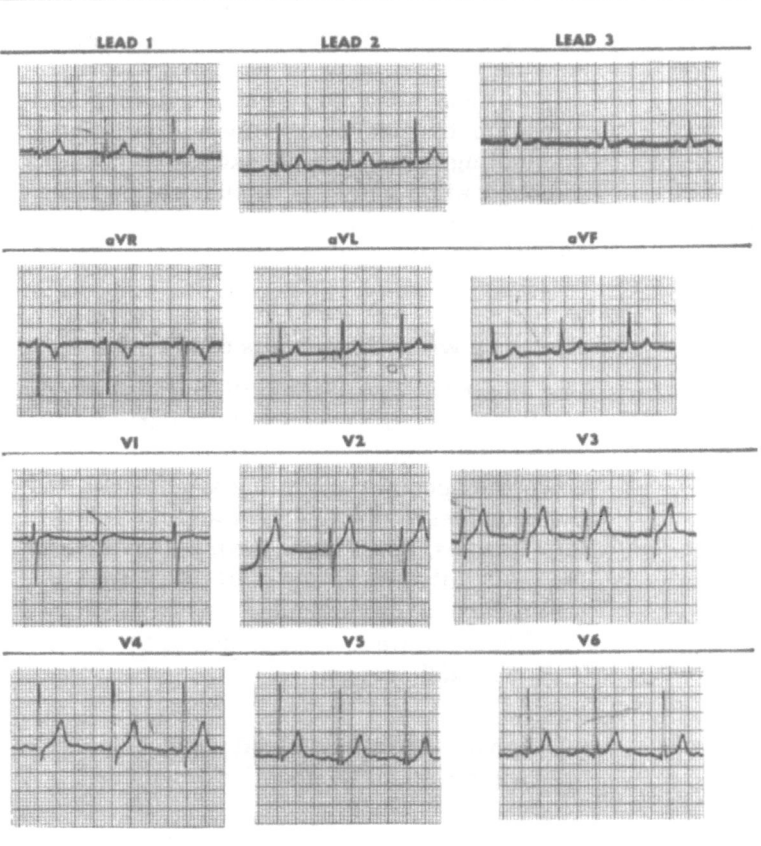

Figure 8.1b   The leads of a normal e.c.g.

From this it may be deduced that the P–R interval represents the time of conduction from the SA node to the AV node.

QRS complex. The shape, height and duration of this will depend on the bulk of ventricular muscle, and is normally greater over left ventricular tissue.

ST segment. This is usually iso-electric (on the same line as the other base line components).

Figure 8.1b shows the leads of a normal e.c.g. The P and T waves are seen to be inverted in AVR.

Reading the e.c.g.

(1) Look at a strip from the recording and observe whether the QRS complexes are regular, i.e. evenly spaced.

(2) Look for P waves before each QRS complex and measure the P–R interval. Each small square represents 0.04 seconds. If this is normal the patient is in sinus rhythm (normal value 0.12–0.2 seconds).

If P waves are absent, the recording is of some dysrhythmia, e.g. atrial fibrillation or flutter, nodal rhythm, heart block or sinus arrest. The P wave is upright in all leads but often not in AVR, AVL and V_1.

(3) If the rhythm is a normal sinus one, the rate may be assessed by counting the number of large squares between consecutive QRS complexes and dividing the number into 300. Alternatively the heart rate measured against an e.c.g. ruler which will give an accurate rate quickly.

(4) Look for the heart's electrical axis. This may be done most simply and roughly by observing in which of leads I, II and III the R wave is dominant, i.e. the largest.

The R wave is dominant in lead II in normal axis. In left axis deviation it is dominant in lead I with a large negative S wave in lead III.

Right axis shift will produce a dominant R in III and a large S wave in I.

(5) Observe the height or depth of R and S waves in the ventricular leads. Large R waves over right ventricular leads signify right ventricular (V_{1-2}) hypertrophy, and over left ventricular leads (V_{4-6}), with deep S waves in right ventricular leads, left ventricular hypertrophy.

Measure R wave height in V_1:

R wave in $V_1 > 8$ mV= right ventricular hypertrophy

Measure R wave in V_5 and S wave in V_2:

R wave in V_5 + S wave in $V_2 > 40$ mV=left ventricular hypertrophy.

(1 mV=1 small square or 1 mm)

In the presence of ventricular hypertrophy the association of an inverted T wave is diagnostic of *ventricular strain.*

(6) Look for abnormal or pathological Q waves. Normal Q waves are often seen in left ventricular leads but not usually in right ventricular leads. They may be seen also in leads I and III and AVL. Q waves may however appear in the presence of ventricular hypertrophy. Pathological Q waves are greater than 4 mV in depth and over 0.05 seconds in duration and signify full thickness myocardial infarction in the part of the myocardium under the exploring electrodes.

A Q wave of over 4mV may however be seen in a normal subject over the left ventricle with a tall R wave of over 20 mV.

Generally the deeper and wider a Q wave is, the more significant it is likely to be.

(7) Analyse the T wave configuration throughout the e.c.g. The T wave is usually inverted in normal subjects in AVR and V_1, and in children and negroes in V_{1-3}.

Inversion of the T wave may be the first sign of infarction or may develop after the ST elevation of acute infarction.

It may be seen in association with ventricular strain where a relative ischaemia develops as the hypertrophied muscle outgrows its vascular supply.

The pattern of abnormally inverted T waves is noted and it must be remembered that other conditions apart from ischaemia may cause T wave changes, e.g. peri- or myocarditis, myopathies and hypokalaemia.

(8) The ST segment. *ST elevation* may normally be up to 3 mV. Significant ST elevation occurs in acute myocardial infarction over the affected area and is usually convex upwards. Pericarditis may produce concave ST elevation changes.

ST depression. The ST segment may normally be depressed by 0.5 mV. ST depression of more than 0.5 mV with an upright T wave may be seen in acute ischaemia or during ischaemia produced by acute exercise or digitalis therapy, when its shape is that of a reversed tick.

Some hints as to the recording of a satisfactory e.c.g.

Practical hints in recording the e.c.g.

(1) The patient should be relaxed without muscle tremor or tension in a semi-recumbent position. The electrode wires must be carefully connected to the electrodes according to manufacturers' instructions.

(2) Wrist watches and metallic jewellery adjacent to electrodes should be removed.

(3) Electric blanket warming appliances under or over the patient should be disconnected from the mains, as even when connected but switched off they may cause interference.

(4) Skin resistance should be reduced by using a good electrode jelly. The areas must not overlap on the chest where the use of excess jelly or smearing may give erroneous location.

(5) The machine must be calibrated carefully before recording so that 1 mm deflection is equivalent to 1 mV.

(6) If the chest lead exploring electrode cannot be made to stick to skin because of hirsuitism, small areas of hair on the chest may need to be removed.

Some examples of common e.c.g. abnormalities

Common abnormalities

Dysrhythmias

Atrial fibrillation

In Figure 8.2 a strip of recording in atrial fibrillation is seen. Note the absence of P waves before each QRS complex.

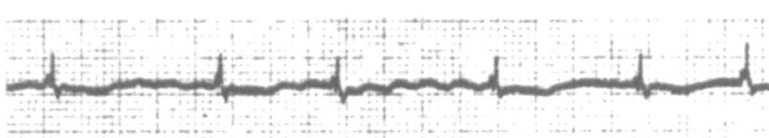

Effect of atrial fibrillation on the e.c.g.

Figure 8.2

The cardiac rate is irregular and fine fibrillary waves are seen in place of the normal P waves representing atrial muscle fibrillation.

Atrial flutter

Atrial flutter waves on the e.c.g. present a more organized appearance than those of fibrillation and a degree of block is present so that each flutter wave will not be followed by a ventricular complex. A four to one block will produce a heart rate of approximately 76 and the heart rate in flutter is usually regular.

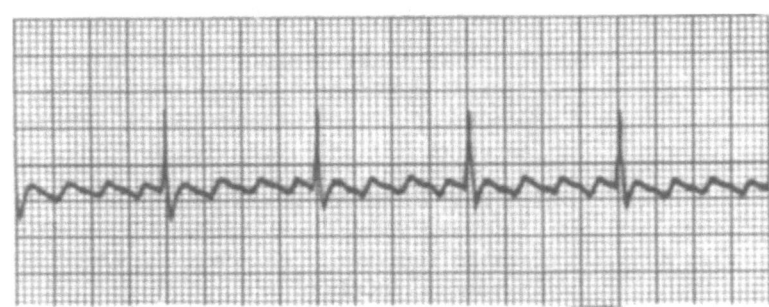

Effect of atrial flutter on the e.c.g.

Figure 8.3

Figure 8.3 illustrates atrial flutter where the characteristic 'saw tooth' flutter waves are seen. There is 4:1 block and the ventricular rate is 74 per minute.

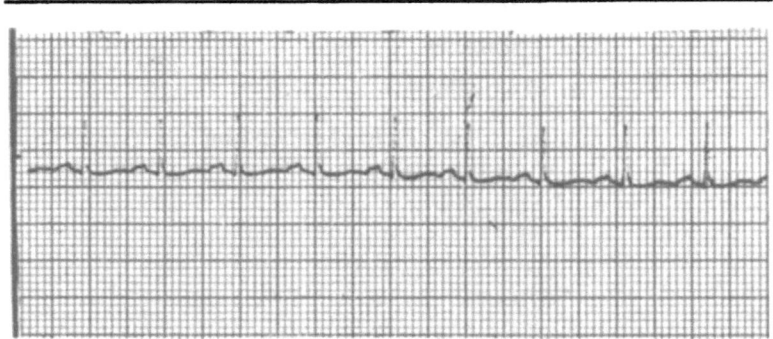

Effect of atrial tachycardia on the e.c.g.

Figure 8.4

Atrial tachycardia

The heart rate may rise to 150 per minute or more and the e.c.g. will show a P wave preceding each QRS complex (Figure 8.4). A degree of block may occur.

Nodal tachycardia

A tachycardia is evident but very often a P wave is not evident or may be seen retrogradely following the QRS complex as in Figure 8.5. A nodal tachycardia will often follow a nodal ectopic.

The nodal tachycardia is differentiated from a ventricular tachycardia by the fact that QRS complexes usually appear normal in shape and the condition is better tolerated clinically.

In Figure 8.5 the P wave is seen to occur retrogradely to each QRS complex.

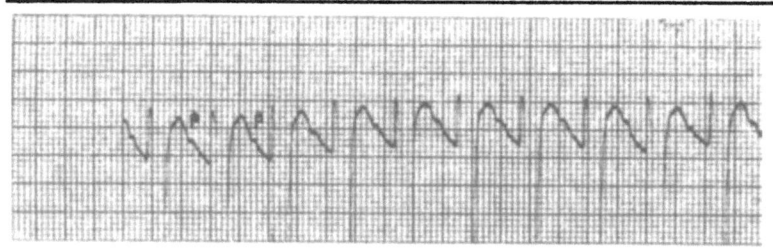

Figure 8.5   Nodal tachycardia

Ventricular tachycardia and fibrillation

Bizarrely shaped QRS complexes occur at a rapid rate (see Figure 8.6) and the condition is very poorly tolerated. If not terminated or treated rapidly this may lead to ventricular fibrillation (Figure 8.7) which is a cause of cardiac arrest and virtually no cardiac output.

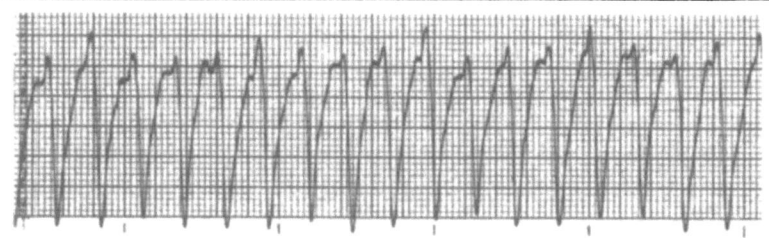

Figure 8.6   Ventricular tachycardia

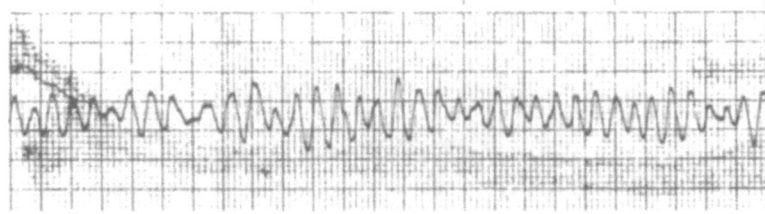

Figure 8.7 Ventricular fibrillation

Ventricular extrasystoles

During a normal run of sinus rhythm a bizarre extra beat appears which has originated in the ventricle and is often followed by a compensatory pause (Figure 8.8a).

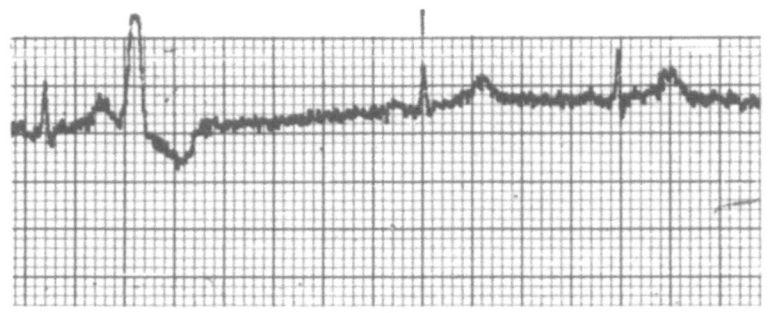

Figure 8.8a Ventricular extrasystole occurring regularly to produce coupling

Figure 8.8b shows ventricular extrasystoles almost falling on the preceding T wave. This is of significance in that it may herald ventricular fibrillation.

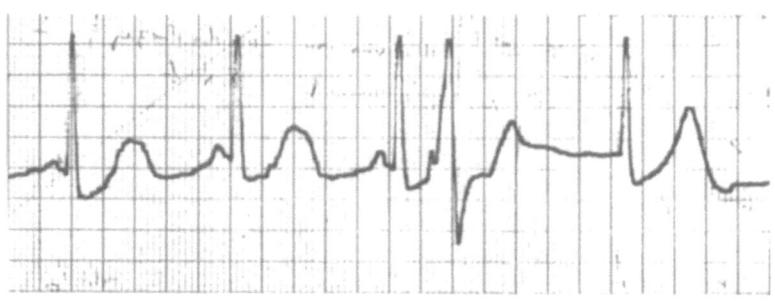

Figure 8.8b Extrasystole falling on the preceding T wave

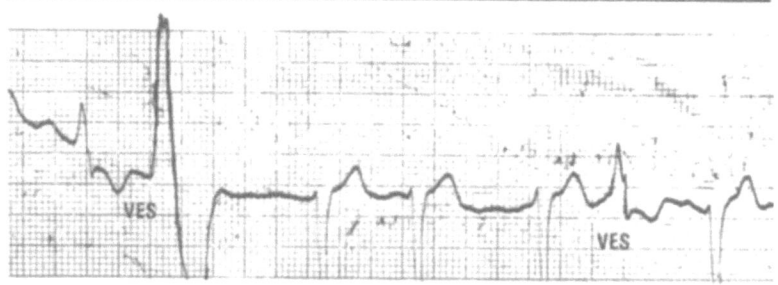

Figure 8.9

Ventricular extra systoles (VES) arising from two foci

The significance of an extrasystole is much more sinister where they are of different shapes, i.e. multi-focal or where the R wave of the extrasystole falls on the T wave of the sinus beat (Figures 8.8b and 8.9) as this may induce ventricular fibrillation. Bigeminal rhythm occurs when a sinus beat is coupled with a ventricular extrasystole, which may not be strong enough to open the aortic valve so that clinically a marked bradycardia may be detected.

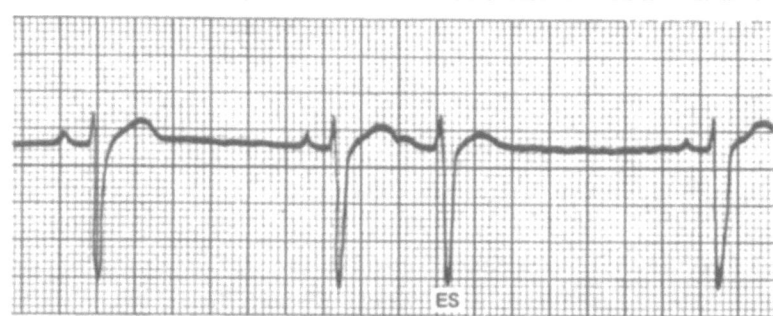

Figure 8.10

Atrial extrasystoles ES = premature atrial extrasystole

Atrial and nodal extrasystoles

Unlike ventricular extrasystoles, these complexes are normal in shape and duration. Atrial extrasystoles occur as early beats preceded by a P wave (Figure 8.10) whereas nodal extrasystoles are not, and if a P wave is seen it is following or retrograde to the QRS complex or may precede the QRS complex and be inverted as is seen in Figure 8.11.

93

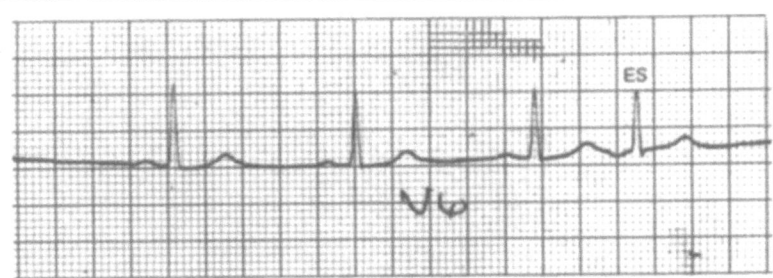

Nodal ventricular extrasystoles ES = nodal extrasystole with inverted
P wave before it

Figure 8.11

Heart block

This occurs in three different degrees.

First degree – prolongation of the PR interval (Figure 8.12),
where the PR interval is seen to occupy seven small squares, i.e.
0.28 seconds.

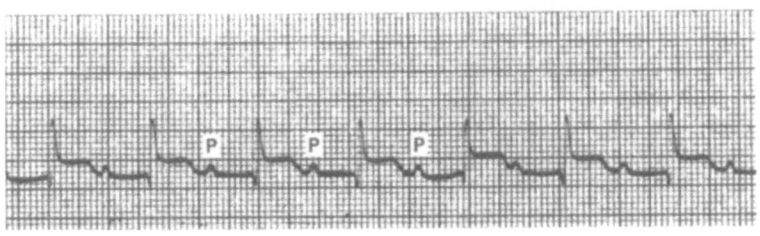

First degree heart block

Figure 8.12

Second degree – the PR intervals increase until a QRS
complex is dropped (Figure 8.13), the Wenckebach phenomenon, or a set degree of block, e.g. 2:1 when two P waves occur to
each QRS complex (Figure 8.14).

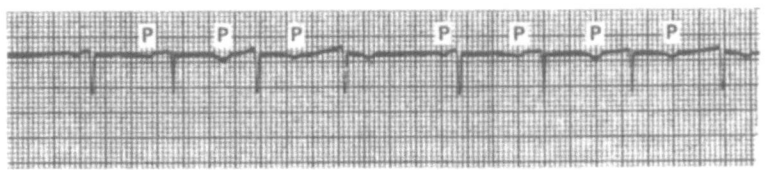

Second degree heart block – the Wenckebach phenomenon

Figure 8.13

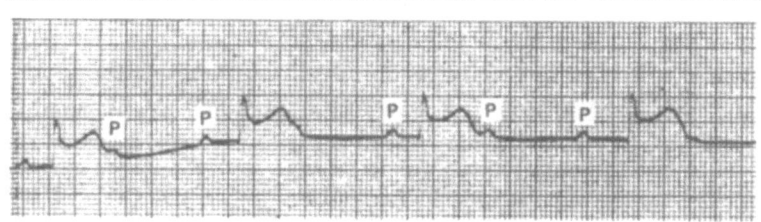

Figure 8.14

Second degree heart block – 2:1 block

Third degree – or complete heart block, where there is no set pattern of P waves to each complex (Figure 8.15). In this tracing long periods of asystole are seen which could lead to loss of consciousness – Stokes–Adams attacks.

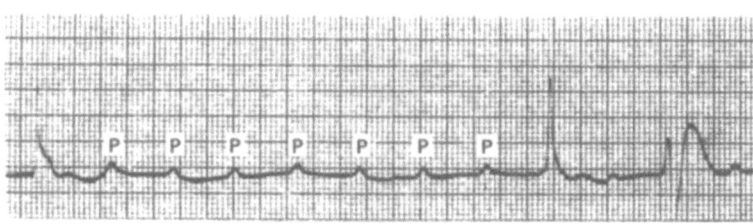

Figure 8.15

Third degree or complete heart block (severe)

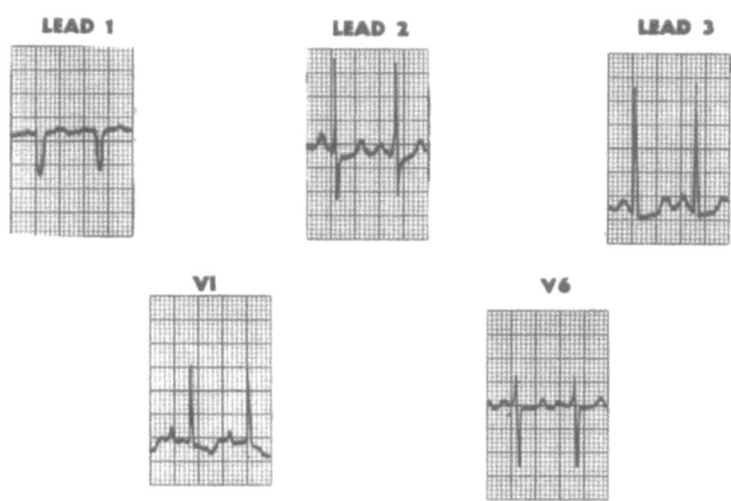

Figure 8.16

Right ventricular hypertrophy dominant R wave and inverted T in V_1

95

Ventricular hypertrophy
Right ventricular hypertrophy

In right ventricular hypertrophy the cardiac axis is likely to be shifted to the right. The R wave in V_1 is dominant over the S wave and measures 8 mV or more (Figure 8.16). The T wave may become inverted over the right ventricular leads V_{1-3}.

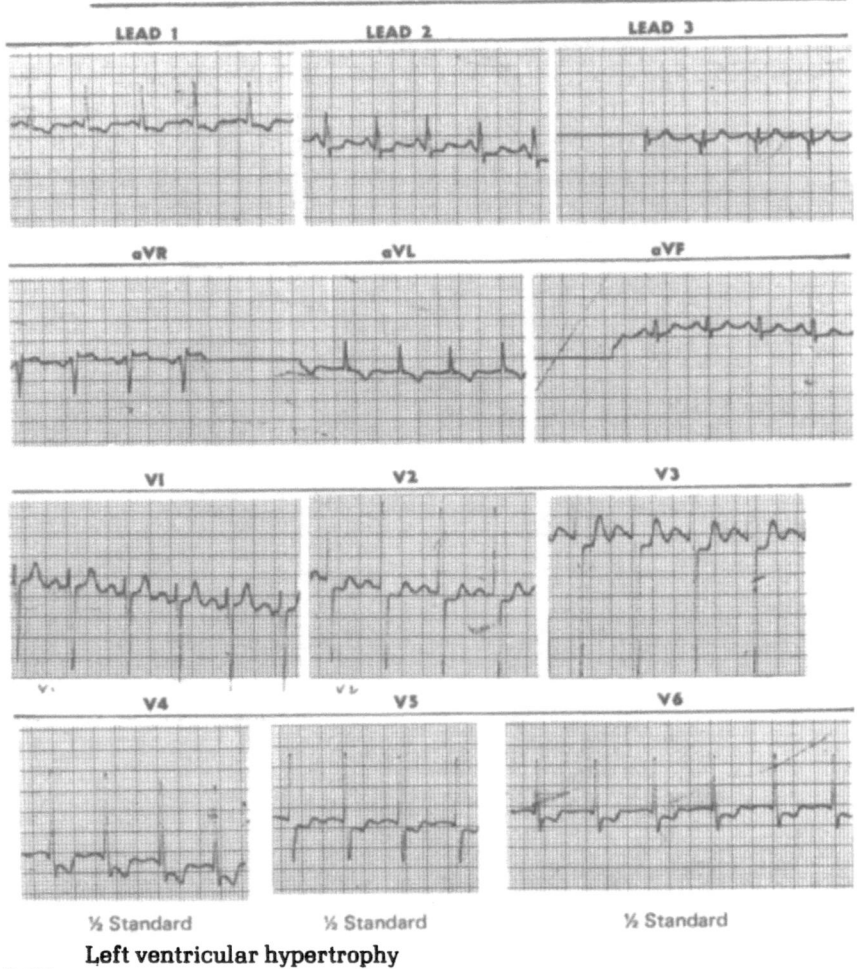

LEAD 1   LEAD 2   LEAD 3

aVR   aVL   aVF

VI   V2   V3

V4   V5   V6

½ Standard   ½ Standard   ½ Standard

Left ventricular hypertrophy

Figure 8.17

Left ventricular hypertrophy

Left axis change is likely. Over the right ventricular leads V_{1-3} there will be a deep S wave with a tall R wave over the left ventricle V_{4-6}. The measurement of S in V_2 + R in V_4 or V_5 will be over 40 mV (Figure 8.17). Note V_{4-6} are half standardized.

$$SV_3 + RV_4 = 30 + 40 = 70$$

The T waves are inverted in V_{4-6} indicative of strain.

Myocardial ischaemia and infarction

Three grades of e.c.g. change are found corresponding to ischaemia, injury, and full thickness infarction.

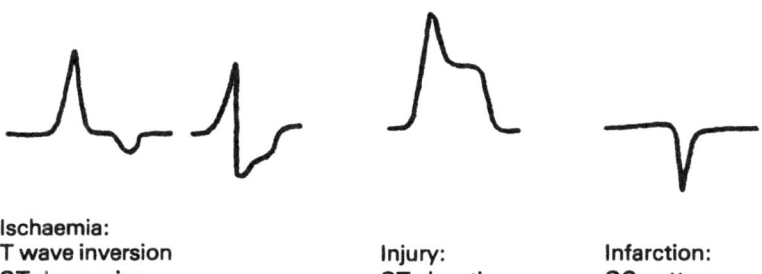

The patterns of varying degrees of ischaemia

Ischaemia:
T wave inversion
ST depression

Injury:
ST elevation

Infarction:
QS pattern

Electrocardiogram changes

Figure 8.18

Ischaemia – T wave inversion or ST depression

An episode of myocardial ischaemia may be manifest as transitory or permanent inversion of the T waves. During exercise significant ST depression may be brought out (Figure 8.19a). These changes are likely to revert with rest. In Figure 8.19b the effects of exercise in producing ST depression are seen on e.c.gs before and after, the test having been terminated by anginal pain.

T wave inversion is frequently seen as a long-term change from an area of old infarction and therefore this finding needs to be interpreted with the clinical situation as to pain pattern.

A patient who has anginal type symptoms may produce ischaemic changes on the e.c.g. which will be circumstantial evidence as to the diagnosis. The e.c.g. may also be normal or show transitory ST or T wave changes.

Sub-endocardial infarction is associated with steep T

97

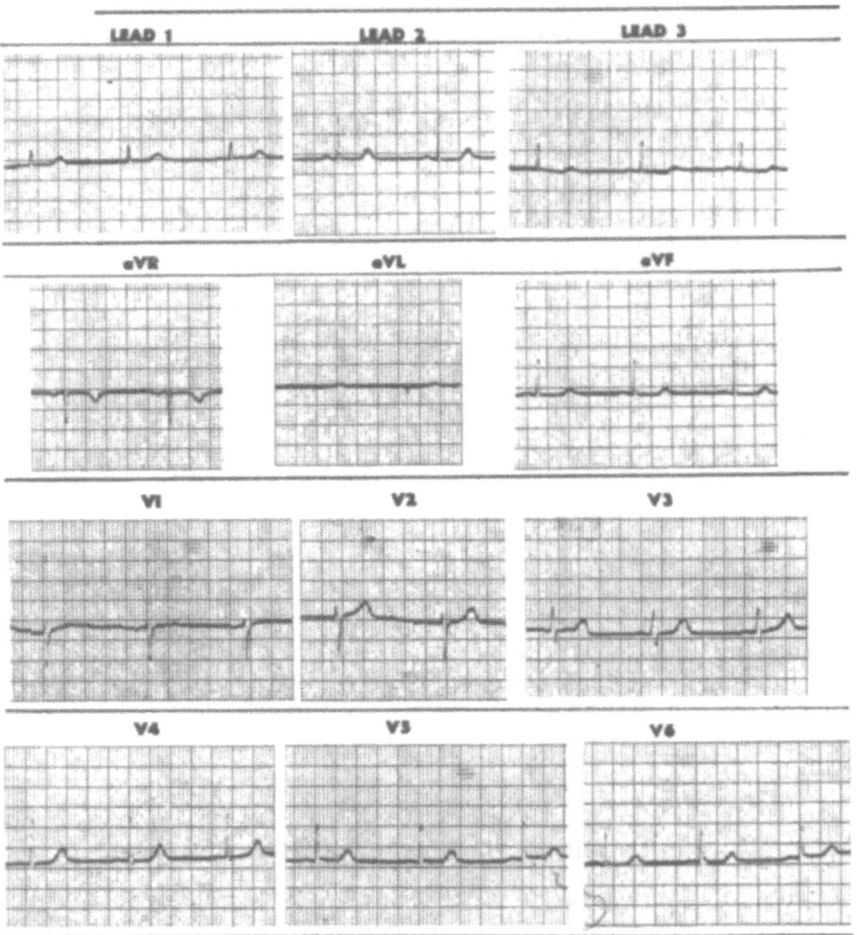

Figure 8.19a

Myocardial ischaemia – resting e.c.g.

wave inversion without Q waves. This is clearly seen in Figure 8.19d This pattern may revert to normal quickly.

T wave inversion may also be found after myocarditis or pericarditis, and in hypokalaemia. Some patients who clinically have had infarcts may only show T wave changes without elevation of the cardiac enzymes. ST depression is found in patients on digitalis and this makes diagnosis of ischaemia difficult (Figure 8.19e).

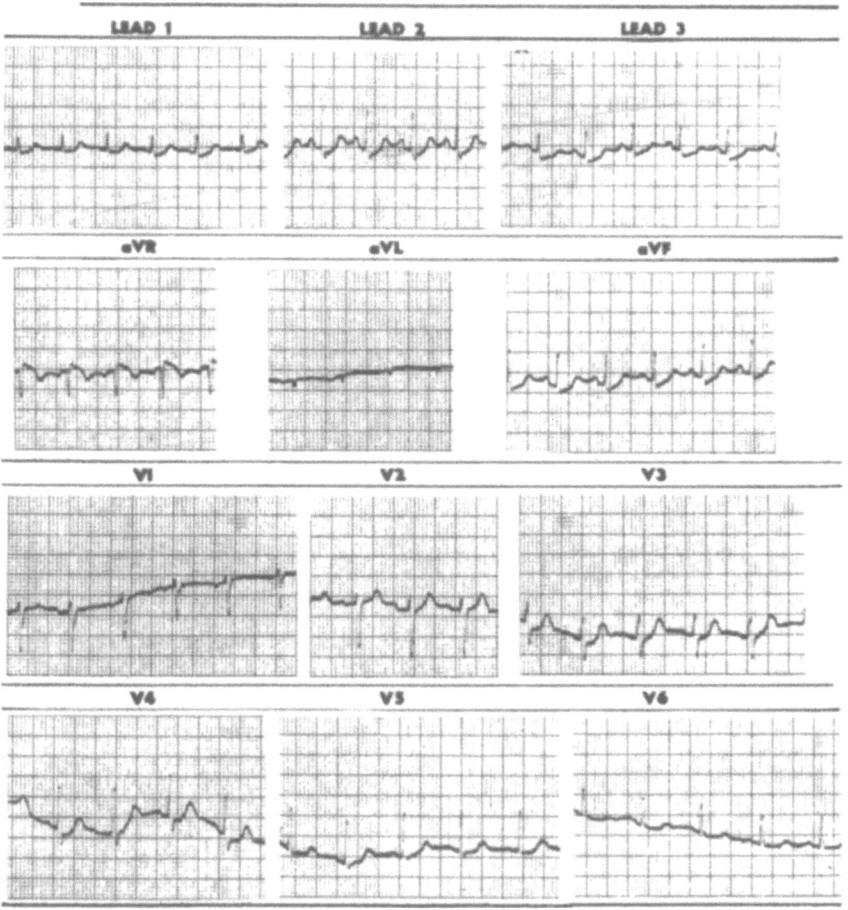

Figure 8.19b Myocardial ischaemia – after exercise. Note appearance of ST depression

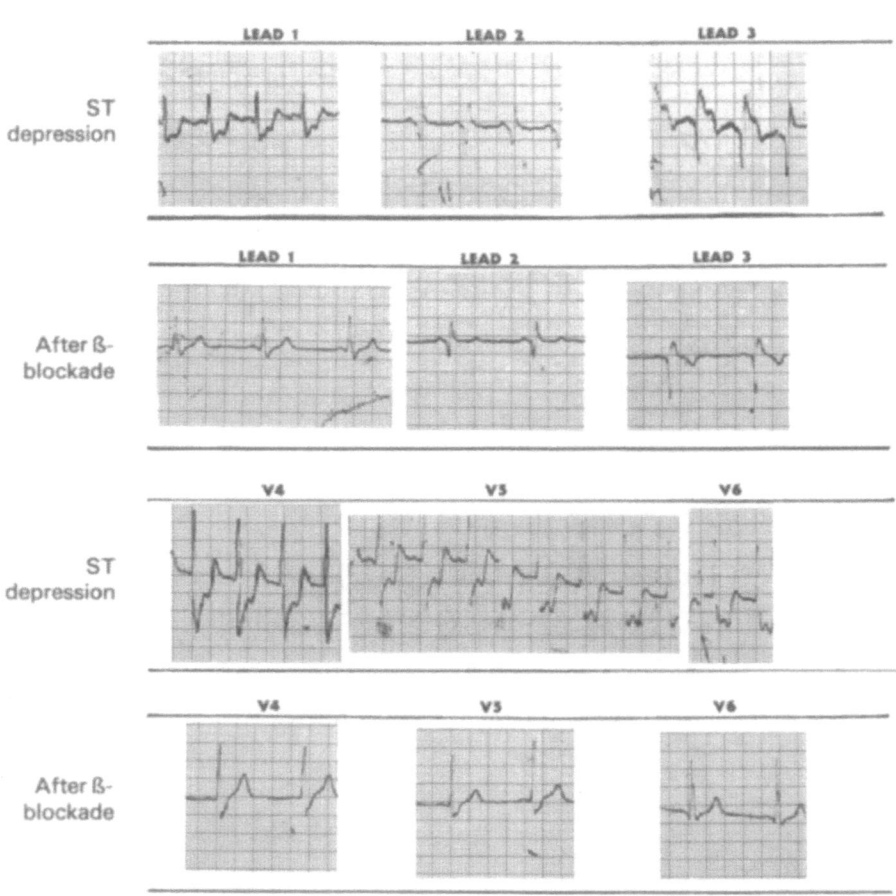

Figure 8.19c   ST depression due to ischaemia reversed by ß-blockade

In Figure 8.19c, ST depression is seen in a patient with ischaemic pain; the pain and ST depression have been abolished by ß-blockade.

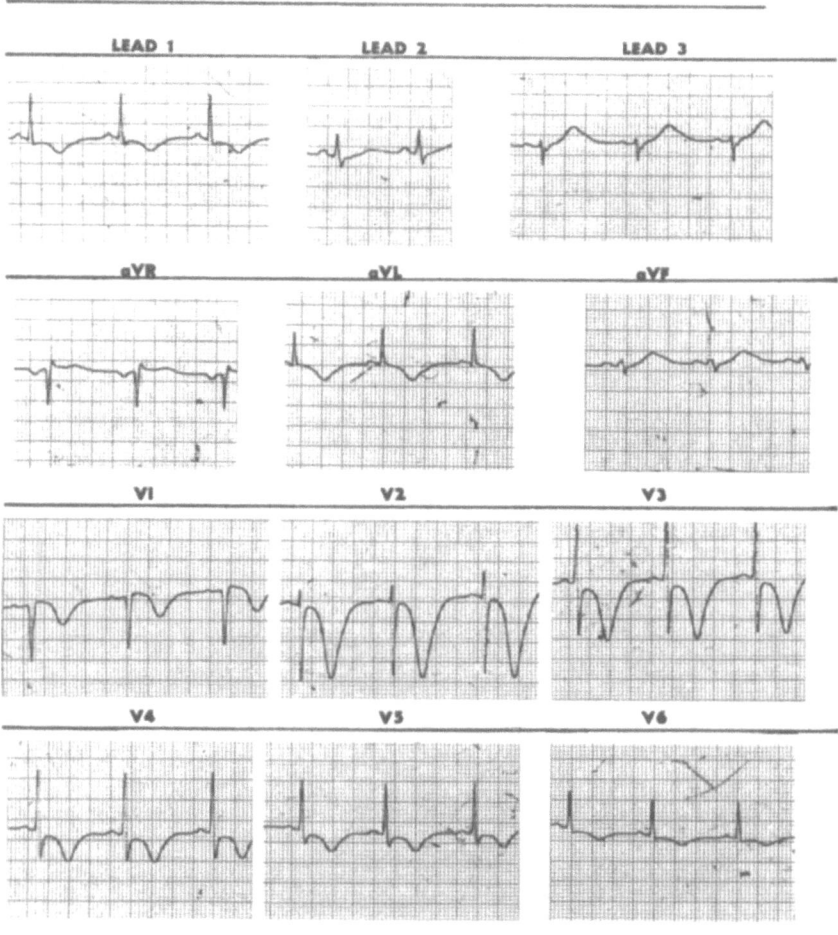

Sub-endocardial infarction note steep T wave inversion without Q waves

Figure 8.19d

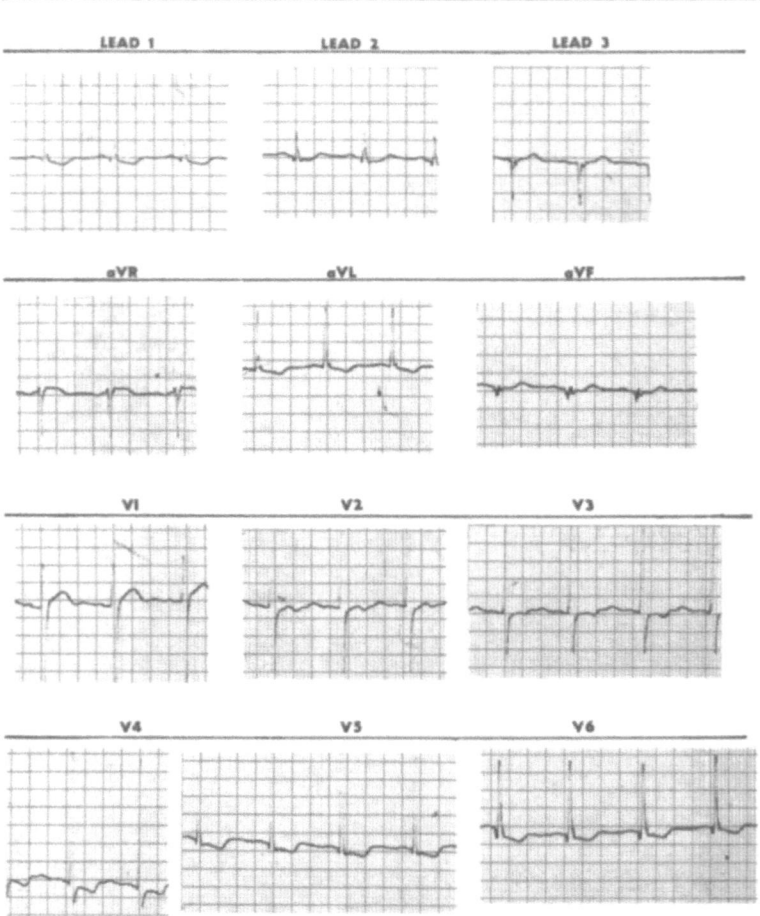

ST depression due to digitalis therapy is seen in I, II, AVL, V_{4-6}.

ST depression due to digitalis

Figure 8.19e

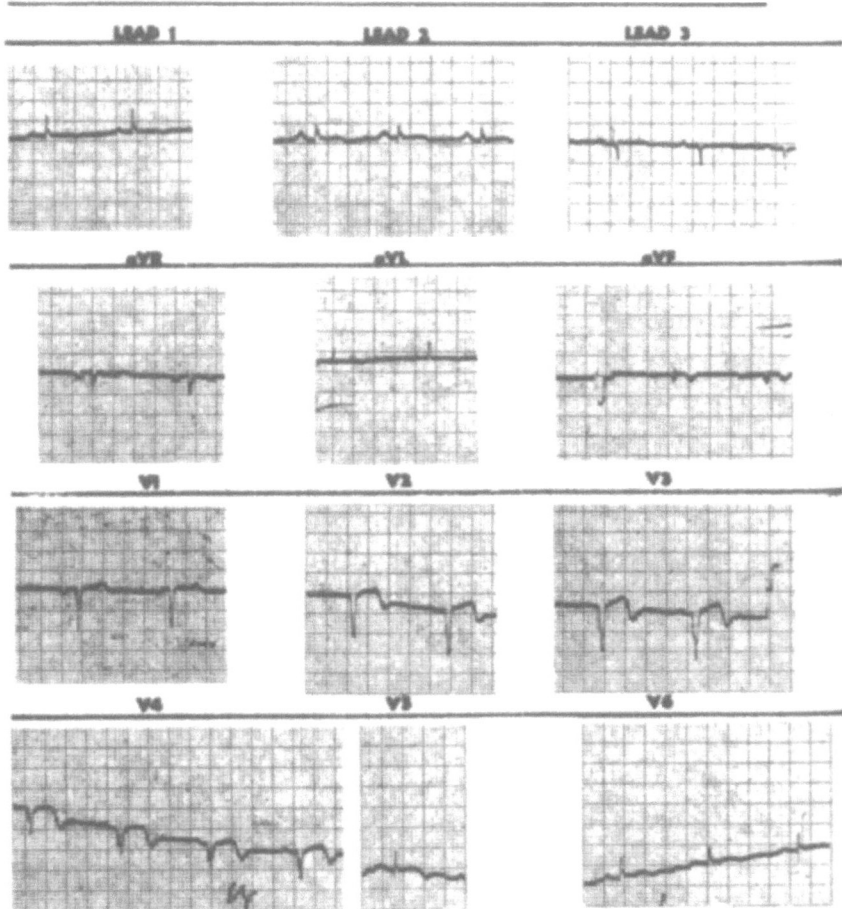

Figure 8.20a

ST elevation proceeding to T wave inversion in anterior infarction

Injury

Actual muscle injury without full thickness infarction will produce characteristic 'convex upwards' ST elevation. This occurs in the initial stages of injury and is followed by restoration to the iso-electric line or T wave inversion. There may be reciprocal ST inversion in the opposite leads. Figure 8.20a illustrates ST elevation in leads I, II V_{2-6} with characteristic ST elevation beginning to invert in an extensive anterior infarct. Figure 8.20b shows classical ST elevation in I, AVL, V_{1-5} with reciprocal ST changes in III and AVF.

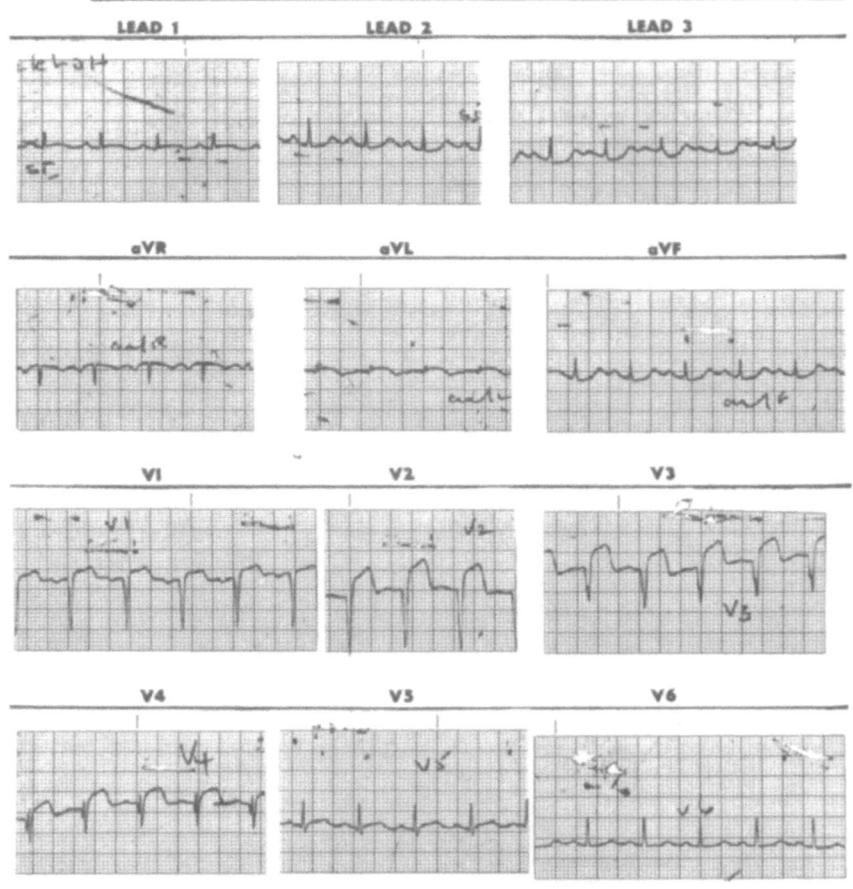

Figure 8.20b ST elevation with reciprocal changes

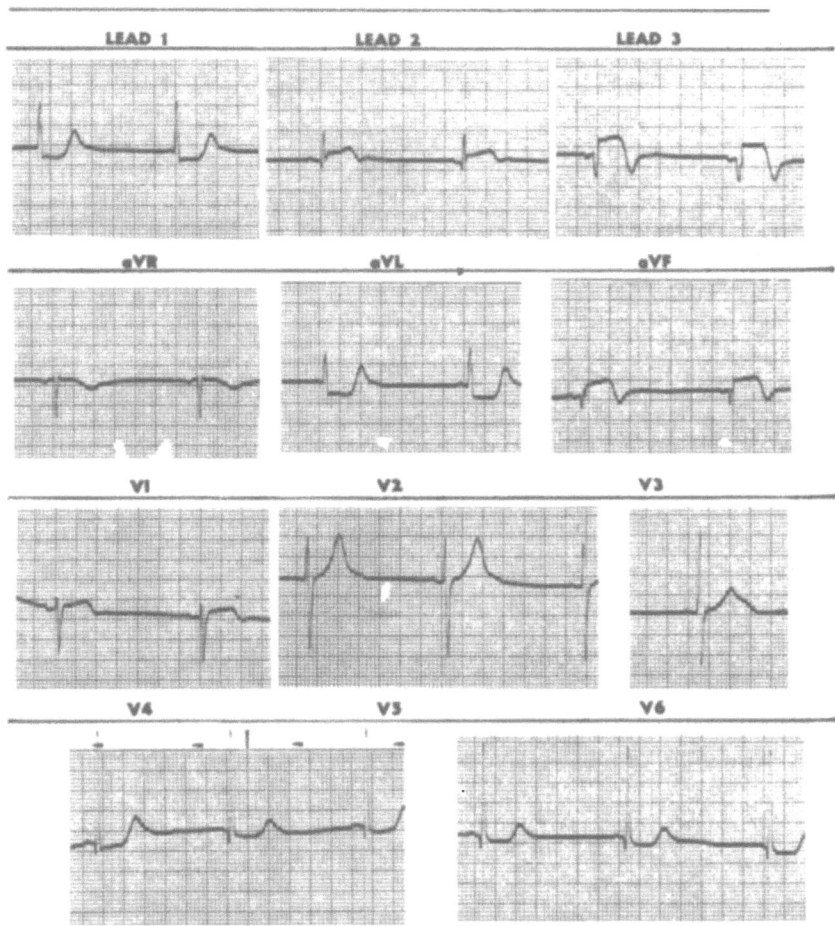

Figure 8.21 Inferior myocardial infarction. Q waves are seen in 2, 3 and AVF with ST elevation proceeding to T wave inversion.

Full thickness infarction

The changes described in ischaemia and injury above are likely to be seen in the area adjacent to the necrotic muscle which is represented on the e.c.g. as a pathological Q wave. Necrotic muscle tissue is non-conductive of electricity and the Q wave represents the negative potential from inside the ventricle. Figure 8.21 shows an inferior infarct with Q waves ST elevation and T wave inversion, in II, III and AVF.

105

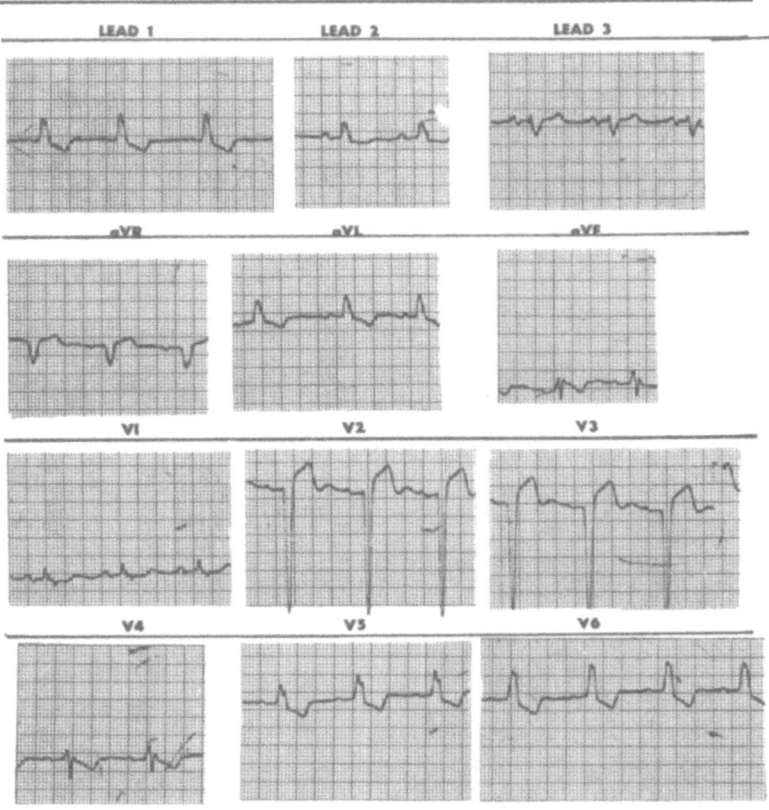

Figure 8.22 Left bundle branch block

Localization of ischaemia or infarction

Areas of
infarction

Infarction is described as:

(a) Anterior,
(b) Antero-septal,
(c) Antero-lateral,
(d) Postero-lateral,
(e) Postero-inferior,
(f) Sub-endocardial.

E.c.g. leads and
infarction

Anterior changes are seen in I AVL and V leads. V_{2-3} are likely to show antero-septal changes and V_{4-6} antero-lateral changes. Posterior or, more correctly termed, inferior changes are seen in leads II, III and AVF and in V_{5-6} if lateral ventricular extension occurs (Figure 8.21).

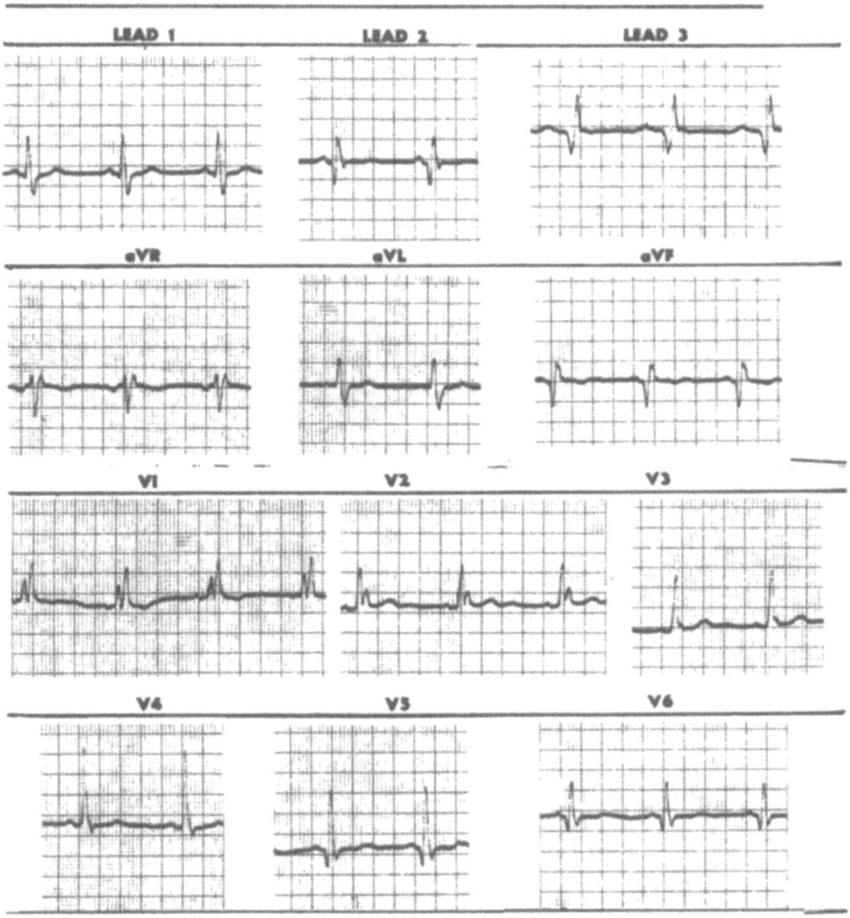

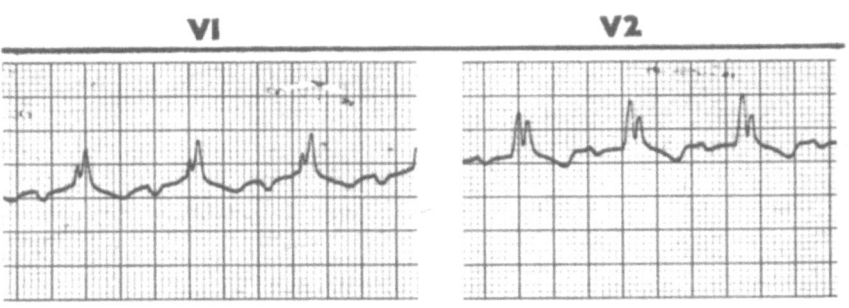

Figure 8.23a Right bundle branch block

Figure 8.23b

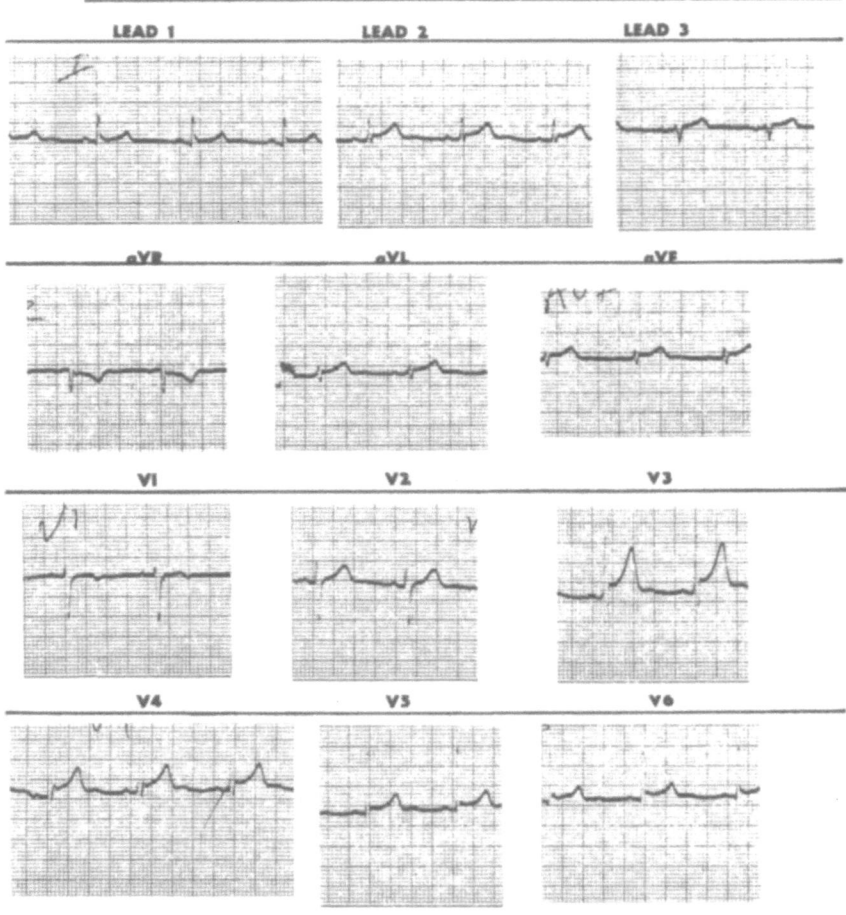

Figure 8.24 Concave ST elevation is seen in I, II, III, AVL, AVF and V$_{5-6}$.

Bundle branch block

Left bundle branch block
In left bundle branch block a bifid and broad QRS complex is seen over the left ventricular leads. The T wave is usually inverted and cannot be taken as being indicative of ischaemia unless a change in T wave pattern is seen on serial e.c.gs Figure 8.22 illustrates left bundle branch block. The QRS complex is characteristically broad and bifid notably in V$_{5-6}$.

Right bundle branch block
In right bundle branch block the QRS complex is M-shaped over right ventricular leads V$_{1-2}$ producing the pattern as seen in Figure 8.23a and b.

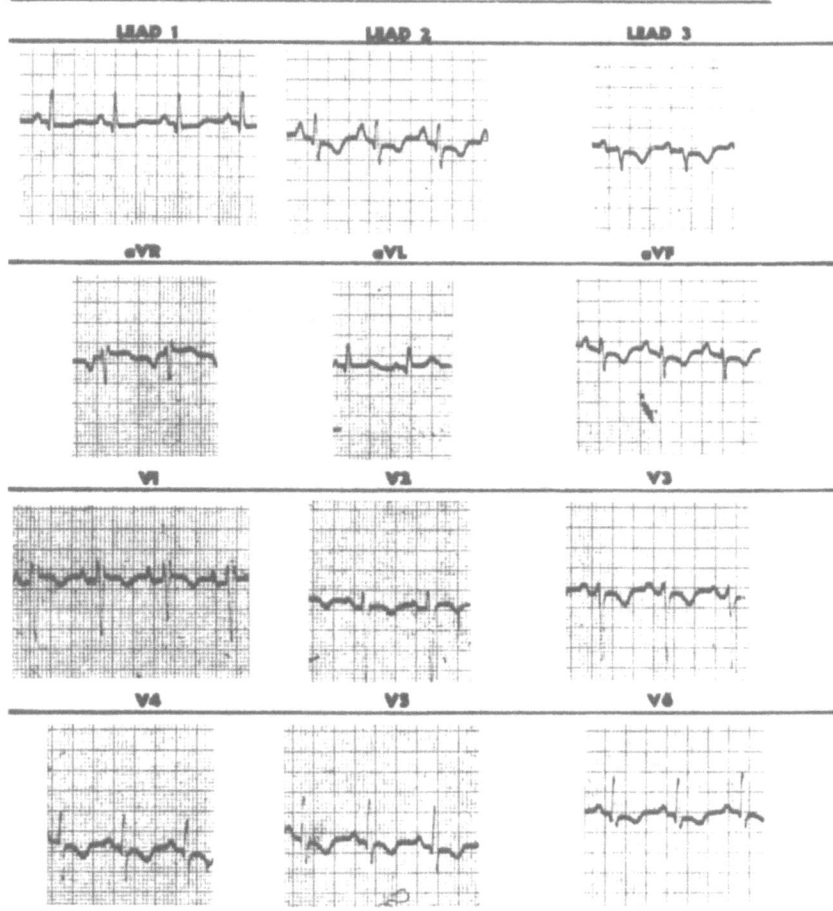

Figure 8.25

Massive pulmonary embolus. Secondary hypoxia has produced T wave inversion over the left ventricle in a case of pulmonary embolism.

Pericarditis

Changes of ST in pericarditis

The QRS complexes show concave upwards ST elevation and these changes cross the boundaries of anterior and inferior localization due to the generalized pericardial reaction (Figure 8.24). ST elevation usually goes on to T wave inversion or resolution to the iso-electric line.

Pulmonary embolus

Pulmonary embolism

In the complete picture, an S wave develops in I, Q in III and T wave inversion in III. In addition the signs of right heart

109

strain may be evident with right bundle branch block and T wave inversion in right ventricular leads V_{1-3}.

In Figure 8.25 the pattern of Q III with T wave inverted in III is seen. There is a peaked P wave of acute right atrial strain. Hypoxia has produced T wave inversion in V_{2-6} and the RSr of right bundle branch block has developed.

Summary

It is important to know not only the value of electrocardiography but also its limitations. Its main value to the family physician lies in assessment of dysrhythmias, assessment of the left ventricle in systemic hypertension and left sided valvular disease, and in some cases of chest pain. A normal e.c.g. does not exclude myocardial infarction nor are ischaemic changes present necessarily in angina pectoris.

The more e.c.gs one performs, reads and reports, the more proficient one becomes and most of the conditions described here are likely to be come across not infrequently by a busy family physician.

⑨ Dysrhythmias

Presenting symptoms – Supraventricular dysrhythmias – Ventricular causes of dysrhythmia – Other dysrhythmias

Presenting symptoms

Palpitations, missed beats, rapid heart beat, rapid and slow heart beat, faintness and lightheadedness, paraesthesiae and pins and needles and exaggerated awareness of heart beat are all common presenting symptoms in the family physician's consulting room or office, and account for a large number of referrals to cardiac clinics for diagnosis.

Anxiety of the patient   Naturally, to the patient any disturbance of the normal heart rhythm is likely to produce anxiety, and patients are often concerned that they are in a state of impending coronary thrombosis. Therefore this type of problem needs careful elucidation, for in the majority of patients referred to cardiac clinics the disturbance of rhythm is a benign one and not significant of any underlying organic disease. There are how- ever some dysrhythmias of great importance that warrant drug medication or the implantation of cardiac pacemakers and accurate diagnosis is of extreme importance.

It has been stated in Chapter 5 that cardiac dysrhythmias account for a significant number of patients referred for unexplained impairment of consciousness. The problem though is of diagnosis, which is not always easy because the patient may not oblige and produce a dysrhythmia at the moment of recording a random e.c.g. Therefore if the problem is severe, it may be necessary to admit a patient to a unit that has

111

24 hour ambulatory e.c.g.s

full e.c.g. monitoring facilities to try and capture runs of a dysrhythmia. A much more successful and reliable method however, is to use 24 hour e.c.g. tape monitoring systems which are now available at most cardiac centres. The patient wears a small e.c.g. monitor with chest electrodes that records continuously the e.c.g. on tape. This enables the patient to carry out normal day-to-day activities which may be important in the provocation of dysrhythmias, and which may be omitted if the patient has to spend 48 hours in bed with a conventional monitoring system. Analysis of the tape of a 24 hour recording takes twenty minutes and will give accurate assessment of any dysrhythmia in that time.

A carefully taken history will often give a good clue as to the diagnosis of a dysrhythmia and the following points in history taking are of value.

Key questions in dysrhythmias

(i) Is the heart beat regular or irregular in timing?

(ii) What is the speed (if this cannot be assessed the patient may tap out the speed with a finger)?

(iii) When does it occur?

    (a) At rest,
    (b) Exercise,
    (c) Relationship to meals,
    (d) With alcohol, smoking or tea or coffee drinking.
    (e) In relation to anginal type pain, and if so, which comes first, the angina or dysrhythmia?
    (f) How long does it last for, seconds, the occasional beat, minutes, hours or days?

(Ventricular extrasystoles are often described as an occasional missed beat when a feeling of lurching or turning over is felt in the chest.)

(iv) How frequently do attacks occur, i.e. how much of a problem is it to the patient? *This is important in determining whether or not to treat the patient.*

The common types of dysrhythmias can be considered in three separate groups, according to origin.

Origins of dysrhythmias

(a) Supraventricular
(b) Ventricular, and
(c) Others.

112

Supraventricular dysrhythmias
Sinus tachycardia

Simple sinus tachycardia

This is a basic normal sinus rhythm at a rate above the normal and is often experienced and complained of by the patient as 'palpitations'. It is found in anxiety states and in states of fear as well or as part of the hyperventilation syndrome when it may be associated with paraesthesiae around the mouth and in the hands and feet, faintness and tightness in the chest.

Sinus tachycardia may also develop as a response to strain on the heart and then occurs as a compensatory mechanism to maintain an adequate cardiac output. This is often found after myocardial infarction, in heart failure, in congenital and valvular disease and in the cardiomyopathies and constrictive pericarditis.

The diagnosis of sinus tachycardia can only be confirmed by e.c.g. but unlike other types of supraventricular tachycardia, the rate varies from minute to minute or hour to hour. The heart rate may be slowed gradually by manoeuvres which stimulate the vagus nerve such as carotid body massage or pressure on the eyeballs, but do not terminate the tachycardia abruptly as may happen in a nodal tachycardia. *Sinus tachycardia when not due to heart failure is well tolerated.*

Treatment

Allaying anxiety

Drug therapy

In states of anxiety, fear and cardiac neurosis, strong reassurance is a key part of treatment and may, with the support of a normal e.c.g. suffice. Simple sedation with a small dose of drugs such as diazepam (Valium) or chlordiazepoxide (Librium) is often beneficial. Occasionally it may be necessary to use a ß-blocking drug such as propranolol (Inderal) to control sinus tachycardia if it is troublesome enough. This drug is particularly valuable in sinus tachycardia due to thyrotoxicosis as it will reduce the other features of sympathomimetic overdrive so commonly seen in this condition. It should not be used without careful consideration if there is any suggestion of heart failure.

When sinus tachycardia is due to organic heart disease, attention must be given to treatment of the underlying condition of which the tachycardia is a manifestation.

Paroxysmal atrial tachycardia

Atrial tachycardia

This condition is most likely to occur in healthy subjects but if it does occur in conjuction with heart disease the prognosis

113

is poor. As in simple sinus tachycardia, atrial support is present so that the condition is well tolerated. It is likely to present at young ages, certainly under the age of 35 or 40 years.

Carotid sinus pressure may well terminate an attack but if it does not do so, it will usually not have any effect on heart rate, whereas a sinus tachycardia will slow it as will an atrial flutter.

Paroxysmal atrial tachycardia may respond to digitalization, but this must be undertaken in hospital with full diagnostic and monitoring facilities. If carotid sinus pressure has not been effective, it is always advisable to refer a patient to a cardiac unit and not undertake empirical antidysrhythmic treatment.

Nowadays other antidysrhythmic drugs are available but their use, or certainly the institution of prophylactic therapy, must be instituted under e.c.g. monitor control.

Paroxysmal nodal tachycardia

Nodal tachycardia
This differs from atrial tachycardia in that atrial support of filling of the ventricles is missing so that it is a much less efficient rhythm. On ecg, the normal P wave to QRS complex relationship is absent. The P waves may be seen to occur retrogradely to the QRS complexes. It is usually not indicative of severe organic disease and may readily respond to carotid sinus pressure, eyeball pressure, vomiting and the Valsalva manoeuvre (forced expiration against the closed glottis).

Well tolerated
Paroxysmal supraventricular tachycardias are well tolerated and sedation and reassurance may suffice until the attack terminates spontaneously. The attacks are often associated with polyuria due to a marked diuresis probably mediated via a reflux from left atrial wall to the release of anti-diuretic hormone. Occasionally the attacks which persist

Drugs or DC version
may provoke anginal type pain or heart failure and drug therapy, e.g. intravenous disopyramide must be given quickly, and if not successful should be followed by termination of the attack by DC cardioversion.

Supraventricular ectopic beats

Atrial extrasystoles
These may be noticed by the patient as a 'palpitation'. They may herald an attack of supraventricular tachycardia and can only be distinguished on the e.c.g. Atrial ectopic beats are associated with abnormally shaped P waves while in nodal ectopic beats the P wave occurs before, during or after the QRS complex and the P wave is often inverted. The QRS complexes usually appear normal in shape.

Treatment is not usually indicated.

Paroxysmal atrial fibrillation

The common causes of this dysrhythmia are:

Idiopathic – causing 'lone fibrillation',
Ischaemic heart disease,
Rheumatic heart disease,
Thyrotoxicosis,
Myocarditis and cardiomyopathies,
Viral infections and toxic states,
Carcinoma of bronchus,
Alcohol.

Atrial fibrillation will give rise to symptoms when it is of paroxysmal nature and the patient passes from normal sinus rhythm to rapid atrial fibrillation. This will be complained of as a 'palpitation' and may be associated with anginal type of pain and lightheadedness or syncope. The pulse and apex beat are found to be irregularly irregular during an attack and some beats auscultated at the apex will be found to be unassociated with a pulse at the periphery.

The diagnosis is confirmed by recording an electrocardiograph during an attack when the QRS complexes are seen to be irregular with a total absence of P waves.

Lone fibrillation occurs in subjects usually over the age of 45 years and the condition runs a paroxysmal course for many years before settling in permanent fibrillation, assuming the condition is purely that of lone fibrillation, i.e. there is no underlying organic heart disease.

Treatment of paroxysmal atrial fibrillation is directed two ways, either to diminish the frequency of attacks or to control the rate of fibrillation when it occurs. Quinidine in a long-acting form (Kinidin Durules) is of proven value in preventing paroxysms, and digitalis is similarly effective in controlling the rate of atrial fibrillation so that the transition from sinus rhythm is less noticeable. As a prophylactic there are good reports of the newer drug, amiodarone (Cordarone).

Electrical DC cardioversion is of no value in lone fibrillation when the return to sinus rhythm is likely to be followed by relapse.

When a patient is in established atrial fibrillation from any cause, treatment is designed to control the ventricular rate to a normal level by the use of digitalis. Paroxysmal fibrillation is best controlled by the use of long-acting quinidine (Kinidin

115

Problems in cardiology

Durules). In a patient who develops atrial fibrillation, and when the underlying cause is a reversible one such as in thyrotoxicosis, mitral stenosis or after alcoholic excess, the patient should be considered for electrical DC cardioversion once the underlying condition has been corrected, when the chance of maintaining sinus rhythm will be high. A patient who is experiencing intermittent or paroxysmal atrial fibrillation, particularly the lone fibrillator, is at some risk from thrombo-embolism arising in the left atrium and must be carefully considered for anticoagulant treatment, particularly of importance if mitral stenosis is present too, due to rheumatic heart disease.

DC version and atrial fibrillation

Paroxysmal atrial flutter

Atrial flutter
The causes are similar to those of atrial fibrillation. Clinically the rhythm is likely to be regular due to the degree of block that exists between the atrial flutter waves and the ventricular beats.

In fixed atrial flutter the rate is controlled by digitalis therapy.

Ventricular causes of dysrhythmia
Ventricular extrasystoles

Significance of ventricular extrasystoles
These represent about the most common cause of the complaint of 'palpitations'. Commonly, they are of benign significance but are more serious if they occur in runs, when they arise from different foci in the ventricles, or when they occur at such timing that the R wave of the extrasystoles falls on the T wave of the preceding sinus beat, for these situations may herald a ventricular tachycardia or ventricular fibrillation.

Symptoms
Ventricular extrasystoles are often complained of by the patient as extra beats, heavy beats, missed beats, the heart stopping or feeling of lurching or turning over in the chest.

They occur frequently in the young and are not significant of cardiac disease but myocardial irritability may be enhanced by certain types of alcohol, particularly following over-indulgence, smoking, in toxic states associated with infections and fever, and in states of anxiety and fear.

At the wrist, the pulse is found to be irregularly irregular and extra beats or the extrasystoles may be heard with compensatory pauses by auscultation at the apex. *Unlike atrial fibrillation, from which the condition must be distinguished, the irregularity disappears with exercise or exertion.*

Patients with this condition are often fearful of underlying heart disease and this fear will generate greater sympathomimetic drive which will accentuate the condition.

Ventricular extrasystoles may signify organic heart disease, myocardial ischaemia for example, and are obviously of great significance when it is demonstrated on e.c.g. monitoring that they precede a run of ventricular tachycardia.

Treatment of ventricular extrasystoles

Reassurance   If it is established that they are benign, strong reassurance of this may be sufficient to allay anxiety, stop patients thinking of and concentrating on the heart beat, and the condition may then resolve. Simple sedation may aid this process and small doses of diazepam (Valium) or chlordiazepoxide (Librium) are the drugs of choice.

Drug therapy of ventricular extrasystoles   If however the ventricular extrasystoles are troublesome and their frequency causes discomfort or fear, it may be necessary to use specific antidysrhythmic drugs for this purpose. The oral drugs that are most useful for doing this and are currently used in the United Kingdom for prophylaxis are disopyramide (Rythmodan, Norpace) at a dose of 100 mg t.d.s. or 200 mg t.d.s., the ß-blockers propranolol (Inderal) starting at 20 mg t.d.s. or procainamide (Pronestyl) starting at 250 mg q.d.s. Disopyramide is the drug of choice currently and its most common side effect, which is not very common, is in causing difficulty of micturition or urinary retention. Very often, after one or two weeks of prophylactic treatment the drug may be withdrawn and the condition does not subsequently recur.

When *ventricular extrasystoles* are associated with runs of *ventricular tachycardia*, prophylactic treatment is essential and will be instituted with the advice of a cardiological specialist. Disopyramide (Rythmodan) or mexiletine (Mexitil) are likely first choices and in this situation treatment will need to be long term.

Ventricular extrasystoles and infarction   The practitioner who finds himself in the situation of seeing a patient who shows ventricular extrasystoles associated with cardiac pain and who may have had an infarction or be threatening to infarct will be well advised to attempt to stop the dysrhythmia by the use of intravenous lignocaine using a bolus dose of 100 mg or by giving intravenous disopyramide (Rythmodan) in a dose of 10 mg over five minutes, before admitting the patient to a specialist unit.

117

Ventricular tachycardia and fibrillation

Ventricular tachycardia and fibrillation

These two conditions are of *grave significance* and if not treated may lead to *cardiac standstill and death.*

In ventricular fibrillation, an emergency, the cardiac output is virtually nothing and it will be tolerated for only a matter of seconds unless it terminates spontaneously (which e.c.g. tracings show does indeed happen), or is terminated by drug therapy or DC shock. Pending specific treatment, output

Management

must be maintained by external cardiac massage. Ventricular tachycardia is associated with some cardiac output, albeit very much reduced, and may be tolerated for several hours by a person with a healthy heart, but very poorly by a patient with heart disease or particularly after myocardial infarction. In any of these situations however, a ventricular tachycardia should be *terminated as a matter of urgency* either by giving drugs such as intravenous lignocaine or disopyramide or by DC cardioversion. The distinction between a supraventricular and ventricular tachycardia is important, for a patient with a supraventricular tachycardia may tolerate the condition for 48 hours and conservative treatment may be indicated (unless it follows myocardial infarction when the condition should be

Significance of ventricular tachycardia

terminated sooner rather than later by either drugs or DC version). Ventricular tachycardia is always ominous and justifies urgent treatment either by drugs or DC shock.

Other dysrhythmias

The sick sinus syndrome (tachy-brady syndrome)

Alternating tachycardia and bradycardia

This is a not uncommon cause of palpitation when the patient alternates between runs of supra ventricular tachycardia and bradycardia due to sinus arrest or delay. It is usually due to disease of the sino-atrial node and treatment is not easy. The patient may complain of both tachycardia and bradycardia with faintness, syncope, breathlessness and angina.

Therapeutic problem

The problem in treatment is that the drugs used to control a tachycardia may in turn provoke profound bradycardia and vice versa. A drug such as long-acting isoprenaline (Saventrine), used to quicken the heart rate, may cause tachycardia.

The decision to treat or not has to be made on the severity of symptoms, and if they are severe and associated with fainting and syncope, an antidysrhythmic drug such as propranolol (Inderal) acebutalol (Sectral) or disopyramide (Rythmodan) should be used in conjunction with a demand pacemaker which will function when the heart rate falls to a critical level.

Dysrhythmias

Heart block

Management
of heart block

Permanent
pacemaker

Drug therapy
of heart block

This may be intermittent and therefore cause palpitations when the normal rate falls to a slow one due to the ventricles taking over their own rhythm originating at ventricular level. These ventricular beats may be felt as heavy beats.

The decision as to how to treat heart block is made on the severity of the condition. A patient who has complete heart block with syncopal attacks or periods of impaired consciousness must be referred for implantation of a permanent electronic pacemaking system. If the block is intermittent, a demand type of pacemaker will be used, i.e. one that is only activated when the heart rate falls below a critical ventricular rate.

If the condition is less severe, and there is no impairment of consciousness, it may be reasonable to give no treatment at all or to use a drug to stimulate the ventricular rate; the drug of choice is likely to be isoprenaline in its long-acting form (Saventrine), at an initial dose of 30 mg eight-hourly. The tremor that this drug may cause may be counteracted by the use of a small dose of diazepam.

Sinus arrest

Bradycardia
due to sinus
arrest

Sudden
death

This condition may present as a palpitation and is associated with marked bradycardia of irregularly irregular type. It is due to delay or absence of activation from the sino-atrial node, and the e.c.g. will show long periods of asystole with no P waves. The condition is important and probably accounts for many cases of sudden death that are brought in to hospital accident and emergency departments already dead.

Atropine (intravenous 0.6 mg) may be effective but cannot be used long-term and oral atropine-like drugs are ineffective. Long-acting isoprenaline (Saventrine) is worth trying to speed the ventricular rate, or the patient referred for permanent pacemaking.

Summary

Palpitations are usually due to a disorder of cardiac rhythm but are often benign. Diagnosis of the exact type of dysrhythmia will often need referral to a cardiac unit. The rate of a supraventricular tachycardia can usually be controlled by the use of digitalis (digoxin), but prevention and termination of an attack

119

will need other types of drug, e.g. disopyramide (Rythmodan), practolol intravenously (the only use for it now in the United Kingdom) or verapamil (Cordilox). Drugs which have membrane stabilizing actions such as lignocaine, procainamide, propranolol and disopyramide will prove the drugs of value in ventricular disorders. The one drug that is most likely to cover both supraventricular and ventricular disorders is disopyramide (Rythmodan). A patient with heart block or sinus arrest experiencing syncope (Stokes–Adams) attacks is very much at risk and needs urgent referral for a pacemaker.

The precipitating causes of a dysrhythmia if identifiable should always be drawn to the notice of the patient, e.g. bending or stooping which may provoke a supraventricular tachycardia. Certain types of alcohol or heavy smoking may cause both supraventricular and ventricular tachycardias.

The correct antidysrhythmic drug for a supraventricular tachycardia may be determined in a cardiac unit by provoking the dysrhythmia electrically via a pacing catheter introduced transvenously, and trying injections of various drugs to see which one is effective in terminating the dysrhythmia. This drug may then be used long term prophylactically.

Alternatively 24 hour tape monitoring systems may be used to record e.c.g. abnormalities under normal day to day conditions.

10 Changing trends in the investigation and treatment of cardiological problems

Investigations – Methods of treatment

There are various types of investigation and treatment carried out in cardiac units with which family physicians may not be familiar and about which they should be able to advise and give information. These are developments that have occurred mainly in the last decade, though some are more long-standing.

Investigations
Echocardiography

This has become a most useful non-invasive method of investigation which depends on the fact that when high frequency sound waves (ultrasound), generated by the passage of an electrical current through a piezo-electric crystal, strike a structure of different density to adjacent tissue, they are reflected.

Method of recording an echocardiograph

A probe is placed on the chest wall and this both generates ultrasound waves and picks up reflected waves which can be displayed on a cathode ray screen or on a multi-channel recorder. By careful positioning of the probe, recordings can be made from different structures of the heart. Moving structures such as valves or cardiac muscle can be recorded on the screen or recorder and will produce a wave form motion. Various parts of this wave form can be analysed and velocity of movement and amplitude of movement measured.

The procedure involves no more to the patient than a normal e.c.g. which is recorded at the same time, enabling timing of movement to be related to the events of the cardiac cycle.

121

Usefulness of
echocardio-
graphy

This method of investigation has become well established as a useful tool in cardiac diagnosis and is of proven value in the diagnosis of mitral stenosis where the severity can be assessed accurately, some forms of mitral regurgitation, tricuspid valve disease, pericardial effusion, atrial myxoma, malfunction of prosthetic valves, and some forms of congenital lesions when not only the absence or anomalies of valves, but also the absence of septa may be demonstrated. Measurement is made of the diameters of various chambers of the heart.

Phonocardiography

Graphic
record of
heart sounds
and murmurs

This is a long-established technique of recording graphically heart sounds and murmurs. It relies on the principle of a salt-crystal microphone placed on the chest wall converting sound pressure waves into proportionate electrical charges which are amplified to a string or mirror galvanometer. By the use of condensers and resistances, both low-pitched sounds and high-pitched sounds are recorded on the same tracing. By displaying the phonocardiogram simultaneously with an electrocardiogram, echocardiogram, or pressure recording from inside the heart as points of reference, it is possible to display normal heart sounds, added heart sounds and murmurs which can be analysed carefully. This technique being non-invasive and therefore atraumatic is of considerable value in elucidating difficult murmurs and heart sounds. It involves little more to the patient than an electrocardiograph.

Vectorcardiography

Recording
forces
generated
by the heart

The normal electrocardiogram records the voltage developed during the cardiac cycle but the vectorcardiogram demonstrates the sequence, direction, magnitude and distribution of forces generated by the heart. Both present, in different forms, information from a single series of electrical events.

Principle of
vector-
cardiography

The method depends on the dipole theory, a dipole being a generator or source of a pair of opposite electrical charges. Vectorcardiography records the electrical field created by a dipole.

An ordinary electrocardiograph measures the forces produced by atrial and ventricular depolarization and repolarization and this produces a scalar record of voltage change. But the process of depolarization produces a difference in electrical potential between two points and this force has direction and magnitude which creates a vector. A vector can thus be represented by an arrow, and the changing vectors during a cardiac cycle by a series of arrows starting at one point. By showing the arrow tips as a series of dots, a vector loop is shown and atrial activity is represented by the P loop, ventricular depolarization by the QRS loop and ventricular repolarization by the T loop.

Value and uses   The value of vectorcardiography lies in the assessment of both left and right and bi-ventricular hypertrophy which produce change in the QRS vectors, because of the increase in amplitude of forces generated by the enlarged hypertrophied chamber with displacement of the loop in the direction of the increased muscle mass. The technique is particularly useful in the assessment of right ventricular hypertrophy. It is also valuable in detecting disturbance of conduction, and because

Localization of infarction   myocardial infarction destroys muscle with loss of depolarization, the non-infarcted muscle vector being unopposed, it is of use in localizing myocardial infarction.

When electrocardiographic change of true posterior infarction, and infarction in the presence of left bundle branch block are not present, vectorcardiography is of value.

Coronary arteriography

This method of investigation has become fairly commonplace in the past decade along with the development of coronary bypass surgery, which it complements.

Method of showing coronary vessels   Coronary arteriography involves the injection of radio-opaque contrast medium either into the aorta to fill indirectly the coronary arteries, or by selective catheterization of different vessels.

The various types of cardiac cathether that are employed to achieve this are introduced into the arterial system most usually by cutting down onto the brachial artery, or less commonly by puncture of the femoral artery. The patient is usually conscious but sedated, and as far as he is concerned the discomfort of having to lie on an X-ray screening table for an hour or so is of more discomfort than the actual procedure.

Risks and hazards   There is a very small but definite risk of death in this procedure which demands extreme care in the selection of patients for the procedure. Deaths that have occurred have almost invariably been in the severely ill and then at a rate of about 0.1%. In one large series, no deaths were recorded in patients with normal coronary arteries.

The morbidity arises from the damage and occlusion of vessels at the site of introduction of the catheter, cardiac dysrhythmias that may occur during the procedure such as ventricular fibrillation or profound bradycardia, both of which in the sophisticated catheter laboratory are not of grave importance. Other e.c.g. changes are seen, such as the temporary inversion of T waves.

Assessing risk

The small but definite risk must be balanced against the clinical indications and information that may be forthcoming and careful patient selection makes the risk acceptable.

Indications

The main indication for coronary arteriography is in the patient who has severe angina which has not responded to medical treatment, thus suggesting a need for coronary bypass surgery. Here it is essential to define pathologically affected vessels before surgery can be contemplated.

In some cases of angina it may be necessary to perform coronary arteriography in an attempt to demonstrate cases of *main stem disease* where the risk to life is considerable and surgery indicated.

Value of coronary arteriography

Coronary arteriography is not a procedure to be undertaken as a pure aid to the diagnosis of coronary disease unless all other methods have failed and it remains essential to made a diagnosis. It is of value in determining the significance of the coronary circulation in a patient with angina and aortic valve disease when aortic valve surgery is contemplated.

Interesting results are obtained from coronary arteriography, and one group of patients has been identified, whose members have typical anginal symptoms and positive exercise e.c.g. tests, but normal coronary vessels. It is thought that this group has disease or disorder of the smaller vessels which cannot be visualized by arteriography but which carries a good prognosis. A further group has been shown in which there occurs coronary artery spasm with anginal pain, the vessels otherwise being normal.

Cardiac catheterization

Methods of catheterizing the heart

The right side of the heart can be catheterized easily by introduction of a cardiac catheter via a vein in the ante-orbital fossa into the chambers of the right side of the heart.

Similarly the left side may be studied by introduction of a

catheter via the brachial or femoral arteries and feeding the catheter retrogradely under X-ray image intensification (screening control).

The information that is obtained by these methods is derived from the measurement of pressures in the great vessels and chambers, and comparing them with the known normal values, from measuring the oxygen saturation of blood taken from different sites inside the heart and vessels and from the injection of radio-opaque medium at various sites, and recording its distribution (cine-angiography). These methods are essential to the accurate diagnosis of acquired valvular disease, congenital heart disease and such conditions as constrictive pericarditis, cardiomyopathies, atrial myxoma and pulmonary embolus.

Indications for cardiac catheterization

Except in the severely ill with very poor cardiac function, the risk is extremely low, and the inconvenience and discomfort to the patient are not great.

Methods of treatment
DC cardioversion or countershock

This involves the passage of large electrical direct current through the chest via two large electrodes or 'paddles' that are applied firmly to the chest wall using an electrode jelly to minimize burning. The electrodes are placed along the axis of the heart, one at the apex and one below the right clavicle. The energy of electrical discharge is measured in watt-seconds. This form of treatment is usually undertaken either as (a) an elective procedure, or (b) in an emergency situation.

DC conversion as an elective procedure

It may be decided to attempt electrical conversion in a patient who has developed atrial fibrillation or flutter or other supraventricular dysrhythmia as an elective procedure. Alternatively a patient who has developed a very rapid supraventricular tachycardia may benefit from its early termination.

Withdrawal of digoxin

If possible it is advisable to withdraw digoxin for 48 hours prior to DC shock to minimize the risk of post-shock dysrhythmias, and to anticoagulate the patient in order to minimize the risk of thrombus formation and embolism when sinus rhythm is restored.

The procedure is carried out under a short general anaesthetic or in a semi-emergency situation, under intravenous diazepam (Valium).

In the correct situation, the morbidity and mortality of

125

this procedure are minimal but the benefits are often considerable in carefully selected cases.

Timing of DC shock

The electric shock is delivered at a time of the cardiac cycle when the heart is not at risk of ventricular fibrillation, i.e. it is triggered to deliver the shock with the R wave of the QRS or ventricular complex and must not fire on the T wave.

Emergency termination of ventricular fibrillation

DC shock treatment is essential for the rapid termination of ventricular fibrillation and ventricular tachycardias when speed is the essence of treatment. In ventricular fibrillation time cannot be spent in giving anaesthesia even if the patient is conscious. Because there are no QRS complexes, triggering the shock is not necessary.

It is likely that in due course most large places of public gathering will have DC defibrillators for emergency use, and the equipment is now carried by cardiac ambulance teams and by some doctors.

Cardiac pacemakers
Temporary transvenous pacemakers

Temporary pacemakers

In certain acute situations, e.g. in heart block following myocardial infarction or in Stokes–Adams attacks due to heart block, it is necessary to insert a temporary transvenous pacing wire via the venous system so that the tip of the catheter is lodged at the apex of the right ventricle. The catheter is

Introduction of pacing wire

introduced into an ante-orbital fossa vein or by a puncture of the sub-clavian vein. Positioning is carried out under image intensification X-ray control and in skilled hands is quick and atraumatic to the patient.

Pacing is initiated from an external box which fires impulses down the pacing catheter of adjustable voltage and frequency. Occasionally, ventricular muscle is irritable during

Irritability of ventricular muscle

and after the introduction of the catheter but this usually passes; but if it remains a problem it may be suppressed by intravenous lignocaine.

If the patient's own sinus rhythm is restored or if a permanent pacing system is introduced, the temporary catheter is then withdrawn.

Permanent pacing systems

Permanent pacing of the heart

Various types of system are used which either deliver electrical impulses to the myocardium at a pre-set fixed rate, or are electronically designed to fire impulses when the patient's own rate falls below a pre-set rate.

126

Positioning of pacemaker

The pacing boxes are fairly small and are positioned under the skin around the axillae, anterior chest wall or anterior abdominal wall.

Pacemaker batteries

The batteries of these pacing units last for two years on average and will need fairly frequent electronic testing to assess battery function.

Electrocardiographic checks are of value in showing that pacing function is adequate and if the pacemaker speeds up or slows by more than two beats per minute below the pre-set rate, there is possible evidence of impending pacemaker box failure. Pacemakers of this type allow patients to lead fairly normal lives indulging in driving and playing certain sports, but care must be taken to avoid strain and trauma on the boxes to minimize the risk of disturbing the transvenous or epicardially fixed pacing wires. Advice about physical activity and travel abroad should be sought from the specialist unit controlling the patient.

Lifestyle of pacemaker patients

Prosthetic and transplanted heart valves

Types of replaced valves

Most family physicians will have in their practices patients who have undergone the replacement of heart valves by either prosthetic mechanical valves, most usually of the Starr Edwards ball and cage type, valves from animals or dead humans (homografts), or valves constructed from patients' own tissues.

In looking after these patients, a large number of whom will be on permanent anticoagulants to minimize the risk of thrombo-embolism, care must be exercised in the detection of changing cardiac murmurs or the appearance of unexplained heart failure, lest there is valve malfunction due to the development of leaks or sticking of parts of the valve.

Other problems that arise are from haemolysis, particularly in the prosthetic ball and disc type valves, and infection causing endocarditis and bacteraemia.

Coronary bypass surgery – saphenous vein bypass grafting

Saphenous vein bypass grafting

This procedure involves removing a strip of long saphenous vein and positioning bypass grafts around sections of diseased coronary artery as determined from coronary arteriography. The number of grafts that are necessary reflects the success of the operation but an 80% abolition of symptoms can be

127

expected in single grafts and a greater percentage may expect improvement.

Indications   Mortality of this operation is not high in uncomplicated cases and the clear indication for this treatment is in the patient who has severe intractable angina which has not responded to conventional medical treatment with the ß-blocking drugs.

There is no definite evidence as yet that the operation improves mortality overall or that it prevents infarction in crescendo angina though much evidence will evolve about these questions.

Type of surgery   The operation involves major surgery using bypass support methods but the patients often complain more of pain in the legs following vein stripping or at the site of the sternotomy subsequently, and this may be a reflection of the success in the relief of their angina.

Summary

There have been many important developments in the investigation of cardiac problems which have occurred and been necessary with the improved scope of cardiac surgery. It is important to know of these as many patients will undergo them. Perhaps the greatest strides have been made in the non-invasive method of investigation, particularly ultrasonic and nuclear medical methods.

11 Drug therapy in practice

Diuretics – The ß-blocking drugs – Other anti-dysrhythmic drugs – Anti-anginal drugs

Prescribing patterns

It is always more satisfactory to form and adhere to simple patterns of prescribing. The following observations are made about the use of drugs in practice from experience that has come during a time of an increasing availability of a number of preparations on the market. Drug prescribing patterns will undoubtedly change but the following views are personal ones which come from the author's own experience in practice. Prescribing certainly presents a problem because of the plethora of products available, and as a general principle it is better to learn to use well one or two drugs from a group.

The diuretics
Acute left ventricular failure and pulmonary oedema

Acute heart failure

The drug of choice in this situation is undoubtedly frusemide (Lasix) in a dose of 20–40 mg given intravenously or intramuscularly. Once this has been given and a diuresis obtained, maintenance therapy should be instituted at a dose of 20–120 mg twice a day, gradually reducing this as improvement follows.

An alternative drug which can be used in acute heart failure is bumetanide (Burinex) which may also be given intravenously (1 mg) and which may prove effective when resistance has developed to frusemide. Use of these diuretics must always be accompanied by potassium supplements in full.

129

Chronic heart failure

Conversion to longer-acting diuretic

Once acute heart failure has been controlled by the use of potent fast and short-acting diuretics, it is prudent to change therapy to a long-acting preparation. The longer-acting diuretics are also used in chronic heart failure and preparations may be used which combine potassium. For example, cyclopenthiazide-K (Navidrex-K) and bendrofluazide-K (Neo-Naclex-K) are effective and widely used. As an alternative, diuretics may be used in chronic situations which have the property of potassium sparing, i.e. they have an action on the renal tubules to promote potassium reabsorption and often make the addition of potassium unnecessary. These drugs are effective long term and spironolactone (Aldactone) is useful as an adjunct to conventional diuretic therapy, and will render potassium supplementation unnecessary. Other potassium sparing diuretics are:

Diuretics and potassium balance

Potassium sparing diuretics

Amiloride + triamterene
Amiloride + hydrochlorothiazide (Moduretic)
Triamterene + hydrochlorothiazide (Dyazide)
Triamterene + benzthiazide (Dytide)

These potassium sparing diuretics have particular appeal in the elderly who may be unreliable in taking potassium supplements. Many doctors are opposed in principle to combination drugs, but a single tablet of diuretic incorporating potassium is both effective and relatively safe. The use of a potassium sparing diuretic will lessen the likelihood of digitalis toxicity in the elderly.

Hypertension

Diuretics in hypertension

When a diuretic is used in the treatment of hypertension it should be a long-acting one. One that is both effective and relatively safe in this situation is cyclopenthiazide-K (Navidrex-K) at a dosage of two tablets each morning.

There is little point in using fast-acting, short-duration diuretics in hypertension since these drugs may cause social embarrassment and interference with daily routine by their extremely potent action.

130

Side effects of diuretics

Diuretics:
side effects

These are listed below.

(i) Dehydration leading to weakness, cramps and thrombosis,

(ii) Electrolyte disorder,

(a) Hypokalaemia with digitalis potentiation,
(b) Salt depletion,

(iii) Diabetes – hyperglycaemia,

(iv) Gout – hyperuricaemia,

(v) Hepatic coma – enhancement and liver failure,

(vi) Marrow suppression – agranulocytosis and thrombocytopenia,

(vii) Vomiting and diarrhoea,

(viii) Provocation of prostatic obstruction and retention of urine,

(ix) Ulceration of lower jejunum and ileum leading to stricture,

(x) Skin rashes and hypersensitivity.

This list appears ominous but although many of these side effects are uncommon they are all important and some of metabolic significance. The side effect that is most common is hypokalaemia in the elderly with digitalis potentiation.

The ß-blocking drugs

In the treatment of cardiac problems the ß-blockers have three main indications:

Indications
for ß-blockers

(i) Coronary artery disease

(ii) Hypertension

(iii) Dysrhythmias

Coronary artery disease

Mode of
action

In this situation, the ß-blockers essentially work by reducing the oxygen requirements and work load of the myocardium by lowering heart rate and cardiac output. This is mainly achieved by blocking the sympathetic drive to the heart which occurs with situations such as stress or exercise, and would normally cause increased work load and oxygen consumption by the heart, with resultant angina.

The ß-blockers have become (together with the use of glyceryl trinitrate) the first line therapy in angina pectoris. The potential prescriber is confronted with a large (at least 18 in the United Kingdom) number of ß-blocking drugs, all of which are effective. It is perhaps best to become familiar and experienced with the use of one or two in different situations.

Dosage of
ß-blockers

It is usually safer to commence treatment of angina pectoris with a small dose of ß-blocker spread out through the day and for this purpose oxprenolol (Trasicor) 20 mg t.d.s. is effective; the dose may be increased and can be converted in time to the slow-release, once-daily preparation, Slow Trasicor 160 mg o.m. which has obvious advantages from the point of view of compliance. Other good alternatives are metoprolol 50 mg b.d. (Betaloc) and propranolol (Inderal) 20 mg t.d.s., both of which may be built up in dosage.

Different
ß-blockers

If heart rate is suppressed to below acceptable levels (i.e. 48 per minute or less) it is worth trying pindolol (Visken) 5 mg t.d.s., which may suppress heart rate less than some other ß-blockers, because of its partial agonist activity. Once the effect of ß-blockers in divided small doses has been seen and established, the larger once-daily regime of longer-acting preparations may be given, of which atenolol (Tenormin) 100 mg o.m., being a cardio-selective preparation, is effective and well tolerated. ß-blockers should not be prescribed in patients with asthma unless it is essential and then a cardio-selective one such as atenolol (Tenormin) or metoprolol (Betaloc) should be used. In the author's experience *atenolol* has been found to be *both effective* and the *most free of side effects*.

Hypertension

The exact mechanism of ß-blockers in reducing blood pressure is not absolutely established but their efficacy is.

Mode of action
of ß-blockers
in
hypertension

After a ß-blocker is given, there may be some initial fall of blood pressure probably due to a lowered cardiac output. But also of relevance apart from the lowered cardiac output is interference with the renin-angiotensin mechanism which is a slower process, with a resultant fall in plasma renin levels.

Most of the ß-blocking drugs have been shown to be effective in lowering blood pressure. Currently the ß-blocker of choice in this situation is atenolol (Tenormin) 50–100 mg o.m. but other drugs that are used and are effective are oxprenolol (Trasicor) 20 mg t.d.s. initially, slow oxprenolol (Slow Trasicor) 160 mg o.m., or metoprolol (Betaloc) 50–100 mg b.d. These represent a personal preference established from observation of their effect in and tolerance by a large number of hypertensive subjects.

If heart rate falls to unacceptable levels, pindolol (Visken) may be tried. In many cases of fairly mild hypertension a once-daily small dose of ß-blocker, e.g. oxprenolol (Trasicor) 20 mg o.m. is sufficient.

Cardiac dysrhythmias

ß-blockers and dysrhythmias

Of the ß-blockers that have been used in cardiac dysrhythmias, practolol was the most useful in all supraventricular dysrhythmias. This can now only be used short-term in hospitals (usually intravenously) and the ß-blocker most like it in antidysrhythmic property is acebutalol (Sectral). This is effective either in the acute situation or prophylactically in an oral dose of 100 mg t.d.s.

ß-blockers also have some effect in preventing ventricular dysrhythmias and ventricular extrasystoles and play a role in the treatment of ventricular tachycardias and ectopic beats. Propranolol (Inderal) has proved effective in this situation. It can be administered intravenously in an acute situation in a dose of up to 1 mg or in an oral dose of 20 mg t.d.s.

Side-effects of ß-blockers

Side-effects of ß-blockers

Bradycardia,
Hypotension,
Lethargy and tiredness,
Nightmares and dreams,
Raynaud's phenomenon,
Diarrhoea,
Cardiac failure,
Bronchospasm,
Mucocutaneous syndrome.

The last-mentioned side-effect was of course the most serious and was associated with practolol which has been withdrawn. Careful exclusion of patients with asthma and incipient heart failure should minimize the two next potentially most serious risks. ß-blockers should not be given to asthmatics unless it is essential, to patients bordering on heart failure without prior digitalization, nor to patients with conduction defects such as heart block.

It is unusual to have to withdraw therapy because of hypertension or bradycardia but pindolol (Visken) may overcome this problem. The other side-effects may gradually diminish with time or may be overcome by changing to a different preparation. Generally, atenolol (Tenormin), has proved the most acceptable and effective of the ß-blockers so far produced.

Other antidysrhythmic drugs

Disopyramide (Rythmodan, Norpace)

Antidysrhythmic drugs

This has rapidly become a first line drug in the treatment of many types of dysrhythmia.

Originally thought to be of value only in ventricular disorders, extrasystoles and tachycardias, the drug is of considerable value in treating supraventricular tachycardias. It is in fact the first choice drug in most intensive care units for most types of dysrhythmia when drug therapy is indicated and may be given in an acute situation by intravenous injection. Oral maintenance therapy is at a dose of 100–200 mg t.d.s. Its main side effect is in causing urinary retention. It has proved a vital advance in antidysrhythmic treatment.

Mexiletine (Mexitil)

This drug is of value in some cases of ventricular dysrhythmia when disopyramide is not effective.

As maintenance therapy following successful termination of ventricular fibrillation of tachycardia it is effective at a dose of 200 mg three or four times daily.

Lignocaine hydrochloride (Xylocard)

Effective in the treatment of ventricular dysrhythmias, particularly extrasystoles and tachycardia, it has to be given intravenously with a loading bolus of 80–100 mg i.v. and may then be administered in an infusion. Overdose with this drug may cause epilepsy.

Procainamide (Pronestyl)

This still has a place in the management of ventricular dysrhythmias for the drug is effective when given orally in a dose of 250 mg q.d.s. It is worth trying when disopyramide and mexiletine are not effective.

Digoxin

Value of digitalis

Mode of action

Digitalis drugs in various forms ((Lanoxin, lanatoside C, or Cedilanid, digitoxin (Digitaline nativelle)) remain the treatment of choice in controlling the ventricular rate in atrial fibrillation when drug therapy is employed. It may also be effective in some other forms of supraventricular tachycardia. Its effect is by depression of conducting tissue with increase of refractory period of the atrio-ventricular node and bundle of His. In atrial fibrillation this protects the ventricle from bombardment with atrial impulses, and the drug is effective as well in atrial flutter. The drug is also effective by its stimulation of the vagus nerve which in turn will slow the heart.

Regimes

Digoxin (Lanoxin) may be given for normal digitalization purposes, with a loading dose in an adult of 0.5 mg followed by 0.25 mg three times per day and continuing this dose until the ventricular rate falls where a maintenance level of 0.25–0.5 mg daily is usual. The drug is usually given orally or intramuscularly but can in an emergency situation be given intravenously.

Hypokalaemia and digitalis

Care must be exercised in both the elderly and young who may be very sensitive to the drug and need considerably lower dosages. The paediatric preparation Lanoxin PG contains 0.0625 mg per tablet and is often in use in the elderly. The toxicity of digitalis is much enhanced by hypokalaemia which can occur as a result of diuretic therapy without potassium supplementation.

Serum level

The serum digoxin level is a useful estimation to check that dosage is in therapeutic range of 0.8–1.8 ng/l.

Side-effects of digitalis

The most common side effects of digitalis are nausea, vomiting and anorexia. The drug may also cause myocardial irritability and preferably should not be administered soon after myocardial infarction. In overdose it can cause supraventricular dysrhythmias and should be withdrawn when a patient on digitalis therapy produces a supraventricular tachycardia, until the serum level can be measured.

Heart failure

Digitalis is of course very effective in controlling heart

135

failure which has been caused by the onset of rapid atrial fibrillation or flutter. This effect is more important than the stimulant effect on the myocardium (positive inotropism) that digitalis has in its role as a pure anti-failure drug.

Quinidine

Quinidine: mode of action

This drug is now used infrequently and has been replaced by other drugs. Its properties include the depression of excitability of cardiac muscle, thus suppressing ectopic pacemakers, prolongation of muscle's effective refractory period which can aid the conversion of atrial fibrillation to sinus rhythm and prevent recurrence. It depresses cardiac conducting tissue and prolongs its refractory period, and by depressing the sino-atrial node it slows the speed of impulse conduction throughout the myocardium. Quinidine in the form of a long acting durule (Kinidin Durules) at a dose of 1 b.d. may prevent atrial fibrillation in paroxysmal or lone fibrillators, and may also sustain sinus rhythm after DC cardioversion. In conjunction with digitalis, it may promote the restoration of sinus rhythm from atrial fibrillation.

Verapamil (Cordilox)

A dose of 40 mg t.d.s. may be effective in controlling dysrhythmias of supraventricular type, but must be used with caution and never in conjunction with or after ß-blockers. It is not a drug to be used freely in family practice. Phenytoin (Epanutin) may be worth trying in a few cases, but in the author's experience is usually unsuccessful.

Amiodarone (Cordarone X)

This relatively new antidysrhythmic drug is now available through hospitals in the United Kingdom. It has been shown to be very effective in the prophylaxis of many types of supraventricular and ventricular dysrhythmias particularly in the prevention of atrial fibrillation. Although microdeposits in the cornea have been reported they rarely give rise to symptoms and usually regress when the dosage is reduced. Normally the dosage starts at 200 mg three times a day, then effective maintenance therapy is usually achieved at 200 mg daily or perhaps on five or six days per week.

Hypotensive drugs

The ß-blocking drugs and the choice of individual ones have already been referred to earlier in this chapter. When there is no contra-indication to their use the ß-blocking drugs are the first line choice of most clinicians, with or without diuretics. The following scheme represents the author's own preferences in drug therapy of hypertension.

First line – ß-blockers.

Second line – add diuretics.

Third line – add hydralazine (Apresoline)
     or prazosin (Hypovase).

Fourth line – consider use of indapamide (Natrilix)
     or clonidine (Catapres).

Fifth line – consider methyl dopa (Aldomet),
     guanethidine (Ismelin),
     bethanidine (Esbatal),
     debrisoquine (Declinax),
     minoxidil (Loniten).

Some comments about these various drugs which either alone or in combination will control most cases of hypertension, follow. Choice of the ß-blockers and diuretics has been referred to earlier in this chapter.

First and second line

See above (pp. 119–123)

Third line drugs
Hydralazine

This drug is currently back in favour after a period of some years when it had fallen into disrepute because of lupus erythematosus which it may cause. In a dose of 200 mg per day or below it is relatively safe from this phenomenon and is very effective as an adjunct to ß-blockers at a starting dose of 25 mg
Hypertensive | t.d.s. In an acute hypertensive crisis a 25 mg dose may be given
crisis | intravenously with a good and smooth effect. The drug given alone may cause an unacceptable tachycardia which will be counteracted by concomitant ß-blockade.

Prazosin

The drug has a similar action to hydralazine, causing diminished peripheral vascular resistance and obviously increasing the effect of ß-blockers in overcoming their adverse effect on peripheral resistance.

The drug is given initially at a starting dose of 0.5 mg t.d.s. increasing this slowly up to 2 mg t.d.s. Sometimes the drug is not well tolerated subjectively, and in too large a dose may cause collapse and sudden loss of consciousness.

In spite of the possibility of the lupus erythematosus phenomenon, *hydralazine has a slight advantage over prazosin* in terms of subjective side effects.

Fourth line drugs

If control has not been achieved with the first three lines of treatment attention should be given to the addition of either indapamide (Natrilix) or clonidine (Catapres), or the substitution of one of these drugs for one already in use. Indapamide is relatively new to the field and its side effects may not yet have been realized. One tablet of 2.5 mg is given in the morning and the drug's action is effective and smooth and seemingly free of side effects. It is a good alternative to ß-blockers in patients such as asthmatics or those with bradycardia who cannot take ß-blockers, and has certainly proved effective when given alone.

Indapamide

Clonidine

Clonidine (Catapres) was for a while a first line choice but does cause some depression, dryness of the mouth, slowing and can, if withdrawn suddenly, lead to rebound hypertension. The starting dose is 0.05–0.1 mg t.d.s. increasing to a total of 0.6 mg daily if necessary. The drug has been of particular value in migrainous hypertensive subjects, a group which may also get considerable benefit from ß-blockers.

Migraine and hypertension

Fifth line drugs

Members of this group are usually added to regimes when control is difficult.

Methyl dopa

Methyl dopa (Aldomet) 250 mg t.d.s. remains the drug of first choice in pregnancy as it is of relative safety and good effect. It has been found to be poorly tolerated by many patients because of its side effects of drowsiness, slowing, depression and impotence. It is surprising that it has maintained such a share of the world market when there are so many better drugs now available. There is little to choose between bethanidine (Esbatal), guanethidine (Ismelin) and debrisoquine (Declinax). These drugs may be added to regimes when control has not been achieved but because they, like methyl dopa, act on the post-ganglionic sympathetic nerve fibres. They will cause marked postural hypotension which may be poorly tolerated. Nevertheless they retain a place in the treatment of resistant cases.

In very severe cases of hypertension when treatment with ß-blockers, diuretics and other vascular dilators have not been effective, treatment may be instituted at specialist units with the most effective peripheral vasodilator, minoxidil (Loniten). This drug has proved very effective in extremely resistant cases. The main side effect is hypertrichosis which can cause severe cosmetic problems. The dosage starts at 5 mg daily increasing up to 50 mg.

Anti-anginal drugs

ß-blockers — The very important role of the ß-blockers as a first line drug has already been referred to. The other first line drugs in the treatment of angina are glyceryl trinitrate (GTN) and Trinitrin (TNT). An alternative drug is similar action is isosorbide dinitrate (Sorbitrate, Isordil). These may have slight advantages in diminishing the chance of headache. Sorbitrate 5 mg may be chewed for quick action.

Free use of GTN — It is important to impress on the patient that GTN or TNT may be used freely with no likelihood of drug resistance developing. The drug may be dissolved under the tongue or chewed for quicker action and can be removed once anginal pain has gone to lessen the likelihood of migrainous headache developing. It should also be used prophylactically to anticipate actions that will be likely to provoke angina such as walking first thing on a cold winter's morning. The drug not only relieves pain but *improves myocardial function* by lessening peripheral vascular resistance.

ß-blockers: contra-indications — If ß-blockers cannot be used or if the patient has not responded to them, nifedipine (Adalat) 10 mg t.d.s. *has proved of enormous value.* The drug is synergistic with ß-blockers and may be effective as well in promoting the growth of collaterals. It has certainly proved a useful adjunct in the control of angina pectoris.

Perhexiline (Pexid) is of value but has the important though rare side effect of causing peripheral neuropathy.

Prenylamine (Synadrin) does not seem very effective and is rarely used now.

It was believed for a long time that a long-acting form of GTN (Sustac) would cause resistance and tolerance to the use of GTN altogether but the drug currently has a place in patients who have angina due to coronary spasm or who have peripheral small vessel coronary disease. The starting dose is 2.6 mg t.d.s. Similarly isosorbide dinitrate (Sorbitrate, Isordil) may be of value in these groups.

Summary

It has always been advantageous to use and know well a small number of drugs. The older cardiac drugs are still of value but the advent of the ß-blocking drugs has marked one of the most important medical advances in decades. The diuretics available are now highly effective and relatively non-toxic. There have been great advances in the antidysrhythmic field.

12 Present and future problems

Changing trends of cardiac disease – Statistics concerning heart disease – Epidemiology and prevention – Logistics

Changing trends

Reference has been made earlier in the text to the changing patterns of cardiac disease over twenty years.

While the effects of rheumatic fever on cardiac valves are still seen and diagnosed in new patients, rheumatic fever is now rare in the United Kingdom and United States. This is due in part to the widespread use of antibiotics in many patients with throat infections, and also in part to improved living conditions. In less developed countries, rheumatic fever is prevalent though this will probably change. The result will be a smaller number of cases of rheumatic valvular disease and the need for surgical treatment will diminish in this group.

On the other hand, the need for surgical correction of congenital heart disease has not changed greatly, and the development of new techniques and methods has brought into the realm of surgical treatment, some previously inoperable conditions. Further to this, some congenital dysrhythmias of the heart may now be treated surgically, although the diagnosis and treatment of all dysrhythmias has improved through technological advances and has been mirrored by the improvement in drug treatment. Drug treatment has become much more specific and less empirical in different types of dysrhythmias. Surgical treatment has been effective in certain dysrhythmias where their perpetuity depends on a circuit re-entry phenomenon. The aberrant pathway may be identified by mapping, and surgically divided to abolish this type of re-entry phenomenon.

Hypertension has become an extremely important condition and its deleterious effects on the cardiovascular system have become recognised and established. Yet there is evidence which would suggest that only a small proportion, perhaps 20%, of men with severe hypertension are receiving treatment so that proper screening facilities will expose this large pool of patients who urgently warrant treatment. This is already beginning to happen in certain areas.

Ischaemic heart disease has become the most important disease of our time, and angina, infarction and cardiac dysrhythmias are its three most important manifestations. They add up to make cardiovascular disease the most important cause of death from the age of 40 years onwards. Not only is the mortality high but morbidity, particularly angina and cardiac failure are of extreme importance.

Cardiac surgery really began to be established in the United Kingdom in the late 1940s. The 1950s and 1960s witnessed the development of open heart surgery with techniques to correct or improve congenital heart disease and replace diseased valves. Temporary and permanent pacing of the heart occurred at this time which also saw recognition of the value of Coronary Care Units.

The major advance of the 1970s has been the evolution of coronary by-pass grafting and evaluation of its uses. There remain several important unanswered questions about it, answers which are likely to be forthcoming in the next decade. It is likely that these answers may encourage doctors into a more aggressive approach to coronary surgery as there is recognition of the value of surgery in certain groups of patients, previously the answer having been unknown. These advances have and will continue, to come at a time of world wide financial recession and stringency which in turn has presented and will present considerable problems of logistics.

In order that one may formulate views as to how these developing problems may best be dealt with, it is important to consider some simple statistics about heart disease and its treatment so that a forecast may be made of the demands on cardiac services in the future.

Statistics

It is certain that coronary disease has become the major

problem in health as it dominates figures of causes of death from the age of 40 onwards. Recognising that mortality statistics from death certificates are unreliable, the 1978 figures for England and Wales show a figure of 31% for all male deaths due to coronary disease. Further, statistics show a marked increase from 1950 to 1970 particularly in younger age groups. There is some encouragement that in the past 8 years the rise has ceased. But as yet there is no evidence of falling mortality figures in the United Kingdom but this appears to have happened in the United States. A look at the table will show that the fall in the United States and the rise in the United Kingdom produces similar figures in the two countries.

		United States	England and Wales
	1968	350	248
Death rate per	1972	323	289
100 000 men	1976	276	272
age 45–54	1977	267	272
	1978	fall	279

These figures pose some extremely interesting questions, the answers to which are not yet available. Epidemiological studies, with particular reference to Social Classes 1 and 2 where there has been a slight decline in death rate, may be of value in providing answers to some questions.

It is of extreme importance that coronary artery disease is the main cause of premature death and the mortality rate in men of 50 or under has doubled in 20 years. In the year 1978 figures show that 42% of all male deaths were between the ages of 35 and 64.

It is difficult to obtain information as to the incidence of problems of morbidity of ischaemic heart disease. In a group of working men, a group that will not reflect a true total national figure because of its selection, the prevalence of angina is reported as being 4.8% in the group aged 40–64. This figure is probably lower than a true national figure.

With regard to congenital heart disease figures can be obtained from rather more accurate documentation. About 8 children in 1000 live births have a congenital cardiac defect and an additional 1.5 per 1000 a congenital type of cardiac dysrhythmia. Of the 8 per 1000, 2–3 will die in the first 4 years of life, half in the first month and 80% in the first year of life. This will leave a figure of about 3 per 1000 who will need surgery for congenital cardiac defects.

143

The need for surgery for elderly patients with calcific aortic disease is a real one and this need has not changed in the past decade and is unlikely to change in the next one.

As cardiological services in a country develop so it is true, do the demands upon it increase and a very good example of this will be seen in the effects that coronary by-pass grafting have had on the attitudes of doctors. The demand for services to provide this facility has risen very considerably as there has been recognition of the operation's value in relieving symptoms. But the demand may rise even more when in addition to this recognition of relief of symptoms, other groups of patients are found to benefit from surgical treatment. Obviously it takes time for knowledge of the value of a treatment of this type to become accepted and for this knowledge then to become disseminated. This in turn puts greater demands on a service. The same has been true of cardiac permanent pacing. If the indications for pacing in the United Kingdom are taken as being the same as the rest of Europe, 75 persons per one million head of population receive permanent pacing systems, yet in Germany the figure is 170 per million. This is due largely to the fact that the development of cardiac services in the United Kingdom has been patchy and that many patients who should have permanent pacing systems have not been recognised. This situation is one that is likely to change as the aim of providing a good standard of cardiological service is reached through the appointment in all regions of physicians with a special knowledge of cardiac problems, and by the education of family physicians as to the recognition of the presenting features of complete heart block and the clear indications for permanent pacing.

But this development of service is an expensive one which puts an increasing call on resources.

The same may be true of the Coronary Care Unit, the value of which has been challenged by some authorities. But it is important to remember the high mortality that occurs in the first 2 hours after infarction, about 50%, and that many of these deaths are due to electrical instability which may occur as the result of a relatively small coronary occlusion or area of ischaemia or infarction. Many of these deaths could be avoided by urgent treatment with the correct equipment in the correct situation. Many deaths are avoided by the use of anti-dysrhythmic drugs, temporary cardiac pacing and DC cardioversion. But the overall reduction in mortality of myocardial infarction may seem to have been disappointing. This disappointment has arisen because of the unnecessary length of time it takes for patients to be admitted to a Coronary Care Unit, an average time of about 6 hours. What is essential if acute Coronary Care Units are to realise their value, is to lower the duration of post-infarct to admission time into the first 2 hours. This has been achieved to some extent by the use of mobile resuscitation teams which can go out quickly, to a home, treat and bring patients in to a Coronary Care Unit quickly. This type of system is of course expensive in every way. There is evidence which supports the hope that earlier admission will result in a higher incidence of successful resuscitation in hospital.

Epidemiology and prevention

It must always be the aim in medical problems, to prevent illness rather than solely to treat it when it has been established. Prevention must be the aim of every doctor is involved in the treatment of cardiac problems though traditionally time, effort and money have been spent over many years in treating well established pathology.

The falls that have been recorded in mortality rates in some countries, notably the United States, Australia, Canada and the Netherlands, are encouraging but are probably due to changes in life style as well as therapy. It is essential that all doctors involved in the care of patients with cardiac problems should be very well aware of and concentrate on the risk factors which have become recognised over the past few years.

They must co-operate fully in programmes to educate the public, children and adults in schemes to remove risk factors from the lives of the population which is at risk.

There are problems in the administration of prophylactic agents of possible value in an indiscriminate way, to the general population though this may be acceptable to a particularly 'at risk' group identified from a bad family or personal history. Screening for hypertension is one field that is of considerable value and one that must be tackled energetically in the future. There is now no doubt at all that hypertension is of paramount importance in the development of vascular disease and warrants a major assault in detection, diagnosis and treatment.

In addition to blood pressure, a determined attack must be made to make the public aware of the risks of smoking. Nicotine stimulates catecholamine production producing a rise of blood pressure and heart rate so increasing the work of the heart.

Carbon monoxide increases permeability of the vascular endothelium and like nicotine increases platelet stickiness. Many surveys have shown that ex-smokers reduce the risk of coronary thrombosis for compared with a continuing smoker, the coronary thrombosis rate is halved in 5 years and at 10 years virtually the same as that of a non-smoker. Other studies support these figures and suggest that cigarette smoking doubles coronary mortality.

Studies in recent years have provided data for a variety of geographically different populations including a wide variety of culturally, racially and environmentally different groups of people. They show a positive correlation between coronary heart disease, mortality and the intake of energy, total fat and saturated fat. Certain biochemical correlations of coronary heart disease are susceptible to dietary change and it is clear that a prudent diet will be one which avoids obesity and also reduces the percentage of dietary energy from fat to a figure of 20–30% rather than the 42% which currently pertains in the western world.

Further to this, exercise must be encouraged for there is some evidence to support the view of the advantages of physical activity in lessening the likelihood of coronary disease. Fitness, physically, is likely to reduce the risk factors as is fitness mentally.

These factors that have been mentioned, obesity and diet, smoking and exercise, are factors that the individual can influence himself. The detection of other factors such as hypertension, hyperglycaemia, hyperuricaemia and hyperlipidaemia are ones that depend on detection and energetic control by doctors. Therefore prevention and the outlook for improving mortality and morbidity figures for vascular disease depend on education of the population as a whole as well as involvement and education of the medical profession.

There is undoubtedly enormous scope for improvement by study of epidemiology and by an educated and determined attack on risk factors by the general public as well as by doctors.

This raises the question of the importance of biochemical screening of the population. This presents a problem practically, and screening is only available currently to a small percentage of the population.

If one screening procedure is to be in use, it is in checking blood pressure, for the rewards from detection and its control are great.

Logistics of the problems of treatment

The evolution of important advances in cardiac treatment by medical and surgical means has taken place at a time when the world has seen recession and economic problems besetting the western world. That such advances have occurred represents a great achievement and the outlook in terms of prognosis, mortality, and morbidity, for ischaemic heart disease and hypertension are dramatically improved in the past decade.

One particular advance has been that of coronary by-pass surgery, the impact of which is not yet fully recognised. It is likely that with the passage of time in the not distant future, further groups of patients will be recognised who will benefit from coronary by-pass surgery. At the present time, there is unequivocal evidence as to the value of by-pass grafting in patients selected for surgery on the basis of their symptoms. The improvement of symptoms and tolerance of physical work has been shown in patients who have undergone surgery and studies have also shown that symptomatic benefit from surgery is correlated with return to work, and to the original occupation. Accepting this, the cost of surgery to the state or an individual is a small one.

But in addition to the group treated only for its symptoms, sub-groups will probably emerge which will warrant surgery for other reasons, and these groups will probably become defined from special types of stress testing using a treadmill and multiple e.c.g. leads; this may be helped by blood pressure recordings and by combination with thallium cardiac scanning which may demonstrate individual coronary artery disease. Coronary angiography is the definitive test which would aid the selection of the 'at risk' sub-groups but this technique presents logistic problems and cannot yet be available to all groups which warrant it.

Selected sub-groups of patients post-infarction may be identified as being greatly at risk by stress testing in association with thallium scintigraphy. In this group those showing S–T segment changes with exercise have a ten-fold increase in 12-month mortality, and it may be that by-pass grafting will reduce this mortality.

Full facilities for investigating these patients are therefore necessary to identify patients with multi-vessel disease and those vulnerable after myocardial infarction. This is in addition to those who need surgery on the grounds of symptoms.

From this, it can be deduced that there is a need to know the demands for coronary by-pass surgery currently, and one may predict what the demand may become as these sub-groups are identified. This is necessary to ensure that health planning has adequate statistics to base its plans on. If one accepts that surgery for coronary disease is offered on the grounds of symptoms alone various studies have given figures for the potential candidates for coronary surgery per year as between 50 to 150 per million head of population. Perhaps realistic figures for the United Kingdom are similar to those for Australia and New Zealand of 110–180 per million per year, and not those of some 350 per million, the figure for the United States.

Now the figure for Australia was based on the indication for severe angina not responding to medical treatment. If one includes the sub-groups referred to above, which are likely to become identified in the near future, as having three vessel disease or left main stem disease, or being early post-infarction patients who are greatly at risk, the figures for the Australian study are low. However, the most recent figures available for South Australian show an operative rate of 600 per million. But in this area, the availability of cardiac surgery is very high, probably higher than is realistic in the United Kingdom or United States currently, but it may give a clue as to the future demands and need for this very important technique. Predictions have not been based on reliable incidence rates of angina but have been based on the incidence of severe symptoms alone.

If one takes all these predictions, figures for South Australia which may be an indication of what is to come and will be needed together with the current figures which probably underestimate the need, a figure for the United Kingdom of 300 operations per million of population is probably a realistic one. This is near to the figure of 350 per million for the United States. Traditionally in the past, more surgery has been undertaken in the United States, for various reasons, not the least of which has been the unavailability in America of anti-anginal drugs, particularly because of the stringent and tighter control of release of ß-blocking drugs there compared with availability, somewhat more relaxed in the United Kingdom.

It is hoped that this discourse about the needs for coronary by-pass surgery will promote thought into the planning for the future and ensuring that adequate facilities are available to meet demands.

It is remarkable that such advances have been witnessed in 30 years, for cardiac surgery has become commonplace and of low risk in many previously hazardous situations. There are also considerable advances in drug therapy, and the speciality is at an exciting point in its evolution. Administrators and planners must be kept aware of what is and will be needed, so that a basically high level of cardiac care can be maintained in all areas and that centres of excellence will continue to provide a sophisticated investigative service. They must also keep pace with the demands that accrue from the advances established from research and the pioneering of new methods and techniques.

Index